Prenatal Exposures in Schizophrenia

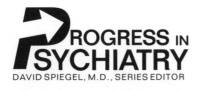

PROGRESS IN PSYCHIATRY

DAVID SPIEGEL, M.D., SERIES EDITOR

Number 56

Prenatal Exposures in Schizophrenia

Edited by
Ezra S. Susser, M.D., Dr.P.H.
Alan S. Brown, M.D.
Jack M. Gorman, M.D.

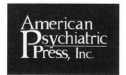

Washington, DC
London, England

Copyright © 1999 American Psychiatric Press, Inc.
ALL RIGHTS RESERVED
Manufactured in the United States of America on acid-free paper
First Edition
02   01   00   99   4   3   2   1

American Psychiatric Press, Inc.
1400 K Street, N.W.
Washington, DC   20005
www.appi.org

Library of Congress Cataloging-in-Publication Data
Prenatal exposures in schizophrenia / edited by Ezra S. Susser, Alan S. Brown, Jack M. Gorman.   —   1st ed.
    p.   cm.
    (Progress in psychiatry series ; no. 56)
    Includes bibliographical references and index.
    ISBN 0-88048-499-3
    1. Schizophrenia—Etiology. 2. Prenatal influences.   I. Susser, Ezra S., 1952-   . II. Brown, Alan S. III. Gorman, Jack M. IV. Series: Progress in psychiatry series ; no. 56.
    [DNLM: 1. Schizophrenia—etiology. 2. Maternal Exposure—adverse effects. 3. Prenatal Exposure Delayed Effects. 4. Virus Diseases—complications. 5. Nutrition Disorders—complications. 6. Autoantibodies—adverse effects.   W1 PR6781L no. 56 1999 / WM 203 P926 1999]
  RC514.P6855   1999
  616.89′82071—dc21
  DNLM/DLC   97-41045
  for Library of Congress   CIP

British Library Cataloguing in Publication Data
A CIP record is available from the British Library.

Contents

Part I
Schizophrenia and Brain Development

Part II
Prenatal Infectious Exposures

Part III
Prenatal Nutritional Exposures

Part IV
Prenatal Immunological Exposures

Contributors

Alan S. Brown, M.D.
Assistant Professor of Psychiatry, College of Physicians and Surgeons of Columbia University, New York State Psychiatric Institute, New York, New York

Peter Buckley, M.D., M.R.C.Psych.
Associate Professor of Psychiatry, Case Western Reserve School of Medicine, Cleveland, Ohio

Pamela D. Butler, Ph.D.
Research Scientist, Nathan Kline Institute, and Assistant Professor, Department of Psychiatry, New York University Medical Center, New York, New York

David Cotter, M.R.C.Psych.
Clinical Research Fellow, Cluain Mhuire Family Centre, Co. Dublin, Ireland

Jack M. Gorman, M.D.
Professor of Psychiatry, College of Physicians and Surgeons of Columbia University, New York State Psychiatric Institute, New York, New York

Hans W. Hoek, M.D., Ph.D.
Chairman, Department of Research, and Director of Psychiatric Residency Programs, Parnassia, The Hague Psychiatric Institute, The Netherlands; Associate Professor, Leiden University, Leiden, The Netherlands

J. Megginson Hollister, Ph.D.
Assistant Professor of Psychology in Psychiatry, Neuropsychiatry Section, University of Pennsylvania, Philadelphia, Pennsylvania

Debbra Klugewicz, M.S.
Research Associate, Department of Psychiatry, New York
University Medical Center, New York, New York

Abbie Lane, M.R.C.Psych.
Clinical Research Fellow, Cluain Mhuire Family Centre, Co.
Dublin, Ireland

Conall Larkin, M.R.C.Psych., F.R.C.P.I.
Medical Director, St. John of God Hospital, Co. Dublin, Ireland

Dolores Malaspina, M.D.
Associate Professor of Clinical Psychiatry, Columbia University,
New York, New York; Head, Laboratory of Clinical
Neurobiology in Medical Genetics, New York State Psychiatric
Institute, New York, New York

Robin M. Murray, D.Sc., F.R.C.Psych.
Professor, Department of Psychological Medicine, Institute of
Psychiatry, London, England

Richard S. Nowakowski, Ph.D.
Department of Neuroscience and Cell Biology, UMDNJ–Robert
Wood Johnson Medical School, Piscataway, New Jersey

Eadbhard O'Callaghan, M.D., M.R.C.Psych., F.R.C.P.I.
Consultant Psychiatrist, Cluain Mhuire Family Centre,
Co. Dublin, Ireland

David Printz, M.D.
Assistant Professor of Psychiatry, College of Physicians and
Surgeons of Columbia University, New York State Psychiatric
Institute, New York, New York

Pak C. Sham, M.R.C.Psych.
Senior Lecturer, Department of Psychological Medicine,
Institute of Psychiatry, London, England

Nancy L. Sohler, M.P.H.
Research Scientist, New York State Psychiatric Institute,
New York, New York

David H. Strauss, M.D.
Clinical Director, New York State Psychiatric Institute, New York, New York; Assistant Clinical Professor of Psychiatry, College of Physicians and Surgeons of Columbia University, New York, New York

Ezra S. Susser, M.D., Dr.P.H.
Chair, Division of Epidemiology, Joseph L. Mailman School of Public Health at Columbia University; Professor of Clinical Psychiatry in Public Health, Columbia University, New York, New York; Head, Developmental Brain Disorders Department, New York State Psychiatric Institute, New York, New York

Noriyoshi Takei, M.D., M.Sc.
Senior Lecturer (Honorary), Department of Psychological Medicine, Institute of Psychiatry, London, England

John L. Waddington, Ph.D., D.Sc.
Professor of Neuroscience, Department of Clinical Pharmacology, Royal College of Surgeons in Ireland, St. Stephen's Green, Dublin 2, Ireland

Padraig Wright, M.D., M.R.C.Psych.
Senior Lecturer (Honorary), Department of Psychological Medicine, Institute of Psychiatry, London, England

Richard Jed Wyatt, M.D.
Neuropsychiatry Branch, National Institute of Mental Health–National Institutes of Health, Bethesda, Maryland

Hanafy A. Youssef, D.M., F.R.C.Psych.
Consultant Psychiatrist, St. Davnet's Hospital, Monaghan, Ireland

Introduction to the Progress in Psychiatry Series

The Progress in Psychiatry Series is designed to capture in print the excitement that comes from assembling a diverse group of experts from various locations to examine in detail the newest information about a developing aspect of psychiatry. This series emerged as a collaboration between the American Psychiatric Association's (APA) Scientific Program Committee and the American Psychiatric Press, Inc. Great interest is generated by a number of the symposia presented each year at the APA annual meeting, and we realized that much of the information presented there, carefully assembled by people who are deeply immersed in a given area, would unfortunately not appear together in print. The symposia sessions at the annual meetings provide an unusual opportunity for experts who otherwise might not meet on the same platform to share their diverse viewpoints for a period of 3 hours. Some new themes are repeatedly reinforced and gain credence, whereas in other instances disagreements emerge, enabling the audience and now the reader to reach informed decisions about new directions in the field. The Progress in Psychiatry Series allows us to publish and capture some of the best of the symposia and thus provide an in-depth treatment of specific areas that might not otherwise be presented in broader review formats.

Psychiatry is, by nature, an interface discipline, combining the study of mind and brain, of individual and social environments, of the humane and the scientific. Therefore, progress in the field is rarely linear—it often comes from unexpected sources. Furthermore, new developments emerge from an array of viewpoints that do not necessarily provide immediate agreement but rather expert examination of the issues. We intend to present innovative ideas and data that will enable you, the reader, to participate in this process.

We believe the Progress in Psychiatry Series will provide you with an opportunity to review timely, new information in specific fields of interest as they are developing. We hope you find that the excitement of the presentations is captured in the written word and that this book proves to be informative and enjoyable reading.

David Spiegel, M.D.
Series Editor
Progress in Psychiatry Series

Introduction

There can be no reasonable doubt that schizophrenia is an inherited disorder. A wealth of epidemiological, familial, twin, and adoption studies cannot be interpreted in any other way. Clearly, the biggest risk factor for getting schizophrenia is having a first-degree relative who has it.

That being affirmed, scientists have recently turned more and more toward the notion that factors other than abnormal genes must play an important role in causing schizophrenia. In the face of strong evidence for genetic etiology, what has motivated this insistence that genes cannot tell the whole story for all patients?

One thing that has *not* turned scientists in this direction is the failure so far to find a definitive chromosomal marker for schizophrenia. The initial enthusiasm that linkage to a locus on chromosome 5 had been established turned into gloom when failures to replicate the finding mounted. This did lead to some pessimism about finding abnormal genes in schizophrenia, but has not changed the conclusion that they must be there. It has always been clear that finding genes for complex and heterogeneous behavioral disorders will be extremely difficult. The rapidity with which linkage for Huntington's disease was found was probably the last time we are likely to enjoy such "beginner's luck." Now we will have to face the fact that psychiatric diagnosis is a complex and difficult process, and this difficulty greatly complicates the problem of correct assignment of individuals to affected versus unaffected groups in genetic studies. We will also have to deal with the age-of-risk problem, with the lack of biological markers for the "silent carrier" state of any psychiatric illness, and with the fact that schizophrenia probably represents a number of interrelated illnesses with different patterns of inheritance. As this is written, scientists are already considering other promising genetic leads, including one on chromosome 6 and another on chromosome 10. Perhaps more promising is the use of genetic techniques that do not rely on linkage, such as association studies. Hence, the search goes on.

Other factors, therefore, have led to the notion that genes are only partly responsible for schizophrenia. As Malaspina, Sohler, and Susser note in Chapter 2, the concordance rate for schizophrenia among monozygotic twins is only about 60%. Most illnesses that follow routine Mendelian rules have concordance rates closer to 100%. Although there are many ways that a genetic disorder could manifest this degree of discordance, the fact that discordant identical twins have a number of objectively determined differences, including the size of several brain structures, suggests that something besides simple inheritance is causing the illness. It is also well known that many patients with schizophrenia do not seem to have any relatives with the disorder—and that despite the fact that patients with schizophrenia may be somewhat less likely to reproduce than the general population, the illness still maintains itself throughout world populations from generation to generation.

Many illnesses are now thought to be caused by an interaction between genes and environmental factors. Some forms of diabetes mellitus, for example, are believed to arise when a genetically predisposed host suffers a viral infection that triggers an immune response in which the virus cross-reacts with normal proteins of the host's own pancreas. Multiple sclerosis is also now believed to involve a similar pathogenesis. As Waddington and colleagues state in Chapter 1, " . . . it may be that the gene(s) predisposing to schizophrenia both code for dysgenesis and confer on individuals some varying epigenetic susceptibility to other prenatally dysgenic factors."

In this volume, a group of very distinguished investigators consider a range of possibilities for "epigenetic" elements that interact with abnormal genes. Several authors consider the possibility that prenatal or postnatal factors may be the environmental elements that "turn on" susceptibility genes. Malaspina, Sohler, and Susser (Chapter 2) provide a number of models by which such factors could play a role in causing what is otherwise clearly a genetic disorder.

Substantial attention is given in this volume to three potential "epigenetic" factors in schizophrenia: prenatal infection, autoimmunity, and prenatal malnutrition. In Chapter 5, Brown and Susser review the evidence implicating prenatal viral infections as known causes of brain disorders. Particularly intriguing is their work that may identify prenatal rubella infection as a risk factor for schizophrenia. Chapter 4, by Wright and colleagues, details the view that another specific infectious agent, the influenza virus, might be of etiological significance in schizophrenia. Partly because influenza virus is not known to directly infect brain tissue, they conclude that "antibodies of maternal origin are elicited in immunogenetically predisposed women by the influenza virus, cross the placenta and the immature fetal blood–brain barrier during the second trimester of gestation, and disrupt fetal neurodevelopment by cross-reacting with brain antigens via molecular mimicry."

The hypothesis that autoantibodies may play a role in causing schizophrenia is also the topic of Chapter 8 by Hollister and Brown and Chapter 9 by Strauss. In Chapter 9, a case is made for the plausibility of an autoimmune pathophysiology of schizophrenia. A number of studies have now shown abnormalities in the level and production of the important cytokine interleukin-2 in schizophrenia. This protein is a nonspecific marker of immune system abnormality. Strauss has also reported very preliminary evidence of antibody to a specific antigen, the 60-kilodalton human heat shock protein, in schizophrenia. In addition, Hollister and her group have implicated antibodies produced in response to Rh incompatibility in schizophrenia. It is unlikely that a majority of schizophrenia cases are caused by or even involve autoimmunity, but studies of this kind may yield insight into the pathogenesis of a subset of cases. Furthermore, with epitope mapping and other techniques, it may be possible to use autoantibodies to trace back to an offending infectious agent.

Malnutrition at one time seemed an unlikely etiology for schizophrenia. After all, schizophrenia occurs in the developed world, where all too much food is available. The recent finding of a relationship between prenatal exposure to malnutrition during the Dutch Hunger Winter of 1944–1945 and subsequent development of schizophrenia suggests that this dismissal should be rethought. In Chapter 6, Hoek and colleagues review this fascinating association, which suggests either that a catastrophic environmental event may be an unusual cause of schizophrenia or that some subtle interaction between genes and a nutritional deprivation may operate throughout the world to influence the development of schizophrenia. Butler and colleagues in Chapter 7 explore the plausibility of the theory that prenatal malnutrition may increase the risk of schizophrenia. So far, it is known that early food deprivation in preclinical samples can cause abnormalities in two neurotransmission systems implicated in schizophrenia—those of serotonin and noradrenaline—and in an area of the brain believed to be affected by the illness—the hippocampus. Preliminary evidence in animals also suggests that nutritional deprivation in early life causes dopamine-mediated behavioral abnormalities.

Central to most of the theories and studies described in this book is an emerging consensus that schizophrenia is a neurodevelopmental disorder. That is, the damage done to the brain in schizophrenia is believed by these authors to originate during fetal life. Further brain atrophy after illness onset may occur in some, but probably not all, patients. In Chapter 3, Nowakowski presents evidence suggesting that, in fact, neonatal brain lesions can lead to behavioral abnormalities that are not expressed until later in life. To be sure, there is still ample reason to consider the possibility that brain atrophy and progressive loss of both cells and function play a role in schizophrenia. Nevertheless, the notion of schizophrenia as a neurodevelopmental disorder caused by a complex interaction between abnormal genes and a variety of environmental traumas has captured the attention of the scientific community.

In compiling this volume, Dr. Susser, Dr. Brown, and I are indebted to all of the authors, who labored hard at the clinic, the laboratory, and the word processor. Our own involvement in schizophrenia research at Columbia University and at the New York State Psychiatric Institute is largely the result of the vision and efforts of our two leaders, Dr. Herbert Pardes, Dean of the Faculty of Medicine and Chairman of the Department of Psychiatry at the College of Physicians and Surgeons, and Dr. John Oldham, director of the Psychiatric Institute. We thank them, our colleagues, our patients, and their families for enabling us to pursue the search for the causes and cures of one of humankind's most devastating diseases.

Jack M. Gorman, M.D.

Part I

Schizophrenia and Brain Development

Chapter 1

Schizophrenia: Evidence for a "Cascade" Process With Neurodevelopmental Origins

John L. Waddington, Ph.D., D.Sc., Eadbhard O'Callaghan, M.D., M.R.C.Psych., F.R.C.P.I., Hanafy A. Youssef, D.M., F.R.C.Psych., Peter Buckley, M.D., M.R.C.Psych., Abbie Lane, M.R.C.Psych., David Cotter, M.R.C.Psych., and Conall Larkin, M.R.C.Psych., F.R.C.P.I.

O ver the past decade, research at multiple levels of inquiry has, through the concerted application of clinical, structural, and functional neuroimaging, neuropsychological, and neuropathological approaches, elaborated fundamentally on previous notions of schizophrenia as a brain disease (Carpenter and Buchanan 1994; Waddington 1993a). From such studies there now emerges a nexus of a disorder characterized by abnormalities of cerebral structure and function, the subtlety of which might appear at first sight disproportionate to their catastrophic personal and socioeconomic consequences. Among the more consistent themes is one of schizophrenia as a disorder of temporofrontal and corticostriatopallidothalamic network dysfunction; however, there endures a vigorous and healthy debate as to whether such abnormalities constitute a "specific" pathophysiology, with perhaps some left- hemisphere preponderance or other alteration in (a)symmetry and putative overrepresentation in males, or are but

The authors' studies are supported by the Health Research Board and the Stanley Foundation.

elements (albeit important ones) among more generalized cerebral dysfunction (Andreasen et al. 1994; Blanchard and Neale 1994; Bogerts 1993; Carpenter and Buchanan 1994; Gur and Pearlson 1993; Harvey et al. 1993; Rubin et al. 1994; Schlaepfer et al. 1994; Waddington 1993a, 1993b; Zipursky et al. 1994).

The vast majority of studies to date have been conducted cross-sectionally on patients with an established (and treated) illness and thus cannot address directly the fundamental issue of when such dysfunction(s) might have arisen, and the extent to which they might have progressed, in relation to overall course of illness. Nevertheless, numerous strands of evidence point to the importance, perhaps even the primacy, of early (intrauterine) events, as articulated in diverse forms of the *neurodevelopmental hypothesis* (Crow et al. 1989; Kwon et al. 1998; Murray and Lewis 1987; Waddington 1993a; Waddington et al. 1995a, 1998; Weinberger 1987).

In this chapter we outline a "readback" analysis of schizophrenia as a route to clarifying both indirect and direct evidence for such an important role for early intrauterine adversity, and then reconsider neurodevelopmental events as the origin of a "cascade" process; this will be in the context of controversies over the extent to which there might exist active disease and disease progression during the chronic course of the illness (McGlashan and Fenton 1993; Waddington 1993b; Waddington et al. 1998).

A "Readback" Analysis of Schizophrenia

Abnormalities of Structure and Function at the First Psychotic Episode

Studies of cerebral structure on magnetic resonance imaging (MRI) have indicated that abnormalities such as enlargement of the lateral and third ventricles and of the temporal horns, with reduced volumes of the (left) hippocampus, appear to be already present at the onset of psychosis (Bogerts et al. 1990; Degreef et al. 1992a; DeLisi et al. 1991); while computed tomography (CT) has recently failed to reveal ventricular enlargement, it has indicated reduction in total brain volume, (left) Sylvian and interhemispheric fissure enlargement, and widening of the frontal and parietal cortical sulci at onset (Rubin et al. 1993). Similarly, frontal lobe abnormalities such as functional metabolic hypoactivity appear to be already present, not only at the first psychotic episode but also in the neuroleptic-naive state, on magnetic resonance spectroscopy (MRS) (Pettegrew et al. 1991), single photon emission computed tomography (SPECT) (Andreasen et al. 1992), and positron-emission tomography (PET) (Buchsbaum et al. 1992).

Such findings are not confined to brain-imaging techniques. Thus, both briefly medicated and neuroleptic-naive patients at onset of psychosis show neuropsychological deficits at least some of which are consistent with (left) temporal-hippocampal dysfunction, although they may occur against a background of broader impairment (Bilder et al. 1992; Hoff et al. 1992; Saykin et al. 1994). Furthermore, first-episode patients, even when they are neuroleptic-naive, show an excess of neurological signs, although these findings are diverse and do not constitute localizing abnormality (Sanders et al. 1994; Schroder et al. 1992). The presence of structural and functional abnormalities already at the first psychotic episode indicates the importance of clarifying the interval by which etiological processes appear to anticipate these findings.

Psychosocial and Neuromotor Abnormalities as Childhood and Infant Antecedents

Much contemporary evidence now points anew to abnormalities of social adjustment among children in whom schizophrenic psychosis is to emerge in early adulthood. These abnormalities variously encompass social withdrawal, emotional lability, and disruptive behavior in a sometimes gender-specific manner. Furthermore, these psychosocial deficits appear to be preceded by neuromotor abnormalities in infancy, perhaps particularly over the first 2 years, which may affect primarily the left side of the body. This overall profile of developmental deviance may show some specificity for infants and children in whom schizophrenic psychosis emerges in early adulthood, as no such profile appears to characterize infants and children in whom affective or neurotic illness is to emerge (Done et al. 1994; Fish et al. 1992; Jones et al. 1994; Walker et al. 1994). Clearly, if schizophrenia is already characterized by developmental deviance over the first several years of life, the search for etiological processes must be extended backward to yet earlier periods.

Variations in Rate of Occurrence by Season, Place, and Era of Birth

There is a generally consistent body of evidence for a 5%–10% excess of winter–early spring births among individuals who subsequently manifest schizophrenia (Bradbury and Miller 1985), which suggests the operation of a seasonally varying intrauterine factor of etiological significance; arguments that the phenomenon derives from an age incidence artifact (M. S. Lewis 1989) have been rebutted (O'Callaghan et al. 1991a; Pallast et al. 1994; Torrey et al. 1990). Although alternative, gene–environment interaction models have been considered in relation to the phenomenon (e.g., Pulver et al. 1992), we and others have found winter birth excess to appear more common among patients without a family history of the disorder (O'Callaghan et al. 1991a; Sacchetti et al. 1992) and, especially for females, among those who are urban- as opposed to rural-born (O'Callaghan et al. 1995b); urban upbringing may be associated with a general increase in risk for schizophrenia (G. Lewis et al. 1992), and this should be juxtaposed with evidence for generally greater early biological disadvantage following urban birth, as reflected in low birth weight and height rather than current levels of deprivation (Reading et al. 1993). Significant coherence between season of birth in schizophrenia and stillbirth rate in the general population (Torrey et al. 1993) further attests to some association with a seasonally varying factor that acts during pregnancy. Although demographic differences among winter-born as opposed to non-winter-born patients are not prominent (Kendell and Kemp 1987), winter-born patients with schizophrenia (but not affective disorder) may be more likely to show structural (ventricular but not cortical) abnormalities of the brain (Sacchetti et al. 1992) and, at least among males, lower electrodermal activity and more negative symptoms (Ohlund et al. 1990).

Important issues remain, such as secular change in the months of patient birth excess (O'Callaghan et al. 1995b) in the face of secular change in season of birth among the general population over the past several decades (Russell et al. 1993) and the enigma of the little-considered autumnal deficit (O'Callaghan et al. 1995b). Furthermore, evidence suggesting late winter–spring birth excess among children with established neurodevelopmental disorders such as mental handicap (Hafner et al. 1987) and autism (Gillberg 1990), a late spring–early summer birth excess among those with dyslexia (Livingston et al. 1993), and some late winter–early spring birth excess among adults with depression or neuroses/personality disorders (Hafner et al. 1987) would imply the operation of a seasonally varying factor or factors that compromise intrauterine well-being in a more general fashion; differential outcomes may reflect critical issues of timing and/or fetal vulnerability to a particular outcome as a consequence of yet earlier, primary etiological events. There is evidence to suggest that some seasonally varying factor(s) contribute to the emergence of schizophrenia through an action as early as the third or fourth month of fetal life (Kendell and Adams 1991).

Essentially all known diseases show variation in rate of occurrence both in time and in space, and specification of such variation usually provides important clues to these diseases' origin and nature; yet such aspects of schizophrenia remain poorly understood. Geographically, it has been proposed both that narrowly defined schizophrenia occurs at a relatively constant rate in socioeconomically diverse locations worldwide (Sartorius et al. 1986) and that the disorder occurs at substantially varying rates in different countries and cultures (Torrey 1987). However, within a rural, socioeconomically homogeneous region demonstrating geographic variations in prevalence, we found morbid risk for schizophrenia to vary with a location index that overlapped extensively with place of birth, primarily among females (Youssef et al. 1991, 1993). Temporally, it has been argued that the rate of occurrence of schizophrenia may have declined over recent decades (Eagles 1991); in the same rural region, we found morbid risk for schizophrenia to be reduced among persons born since 1940, again primarily among females (Waddington and Youssef 1994). These findings appear complementary to data indicating that the influence of urban origin on season of birth is specific to females (O'Callaghan et al. 1995b) and focus attention on early, intrauterine factors that act in a gender-specific manner.

The challenge is to identify endogenous and/or exogenous factors that act in such a manner and which might vary comparably in space and by era. Although such factors are usually presumed to be "environmental" in nature, we have found (Waddington and Youssef 1996b) that variations in rate of occurrence both by place and by era of birth appear to be superimposed on an unappreciatedly high familial genetic loading for the disorder; thus, such factors could be adjunctive to, interactive with, or theoretically subsumable within a prepotent genetically determined process (Waddington 1993a). These issues are addressed more specifically in subsequent chapters of this book.

The Biology of Early Adversity in Schizophrenia

Obstetric Complications

Long-standing evidence that patients with schizophrenia appear more likely to have been born following a pregnancy/delivery that was complicated in some manner (Eagles et al. 1990; S. W. Lewis and Murray 1987; McNeil 1991) would seem, at one level, to reveal a more tangible mechanism by which developmental insult might be imparted to the fetus/neonate; since publication of a chasteningly negative study (Done et al. 1991), additional positive (Gunther-Genta et al. 1994; Heun and Maier 1993; O'Callaghan et al. 1992b; Verdoux and Bourgeois 1993) or at least equivocal (Buka et al. 1993; McCreadie et al. 1992) reports have emerged (see Geddes and Lawrie 1995; Jones et al. 1998). It has usually proved difficult to resist the temptation to interpret the association in terms of a specific causal relationship whereby obstetric complications directly cause fetal or early neonatal damage and hence increase risk for schizophrenia in adulthood; perinatal asphyxia has attracted the most consistent interest as a putative pathophysiological mechanism.

However, the term *obstetric complications* generally encompasses a "mixed bag" of pre- and perinatal adversities, with no particular complication(s) being identified reliably as having any specific relationship to subsequent schizophrenia (O'Callaghan et al. 1992b). It is thus necessary to ask the question of why the pregnancy and/or delivery of individuals who subsequently evidence this disorder appears to be more complicated in so amorphous a manner. Do such vicissitudes simply reflect normal biological variation in obstetric health? While this may in part be so, it cannot be excluded that certain obstetric complications that occur to excess have some basis in yet earlier events and arise at least in part consequent to a fetus that has already been compromised in some manner at, or subjected to a more generalized growth deficit from, an earlier stage in the pregnancy (O'Callaghan et al. 1992b). For example, there is strong evidence that typical (and thus more readily recalled/recorded) perinatal complications such as low birthweight and prematurity are actually more common in women who have experienced possibly subtle (and therefore less readily recalled/recorded) vaginal bleeding in the first trimester (Williams et al. 1991); such threatened miscarriages commonly occur in association with embryonic abnormalities or maternal–fetal immunological rejection (Chamberlain 1991). Similarly, preeclampsia, also an evident complication of the middle to late stages of pregnancy, may derive from yet earlier processes relating to the fetus, particularly fetal genotype vis-à-vis the mother (Cooper et al. 1993). Finally, cord complications at delivery, noted to be prominent in two studies of obstetric complications in schizophrenia (Gunther-Genta et al. 1994; O'Callaghan et al. 1990), may reflect suboptimal fetal motor behavior consequent to neurointegrative deficits arising earlier in pregnancy (Fish et al. 1992; Sival 1993; Walker et al. 1994).

Part of the difficulty in relating the diversity of obstetric complications in any specific manner to increased risk for schizophrenia might arise from the operation of two distinct processes: one may give rise to complications early in pregnancy that constitute antecedents to other complications later therein or at delivery, and that themselves reflect a fetus already compromised by yet earlier adversity related to the etiology of the disorder; another may occur through vicissitudes originating late in pregnancy, in a manner unrelated to earlier etiological events, and may give rise to nonspecific cerebral dysfunction by way of their well-known liability for periventricular hemorrhaging and associated structural abnormalities (Cannon et al. 1993; S. W. Lewis and Murray 1987). In an MRI study (O'Callaghan et al. 1995a), obstetric complications in schizophrenia were associated not with overall increase in ventricular volume but rather with ventricular asymmetry (left > right). The fundamental issue is to clarify the extent to which typical complications identified in middle to late pregnancy might represent sequelae of earlier events rather than pathological insults and to seek clues as to the nature of any such early antecedent factors and their putative relationship to cerebral dysplasia. One clue may be found in emerging evidence for an earlier onset of psychosis among those male (but not female) patients having a history of obstetric complications (O'Callaghan et al. 1992b).

Minor Physical Anomalies

Perhaps the strongest biological evidence for early dysmorphogenesis is an excess in schizophrenia of minor physical anomalies (i.e., slight anatomic malformations) in regions of the body that, like the brain, develop from ectodermal tissue and are structurally codified during the first or early second trimester; the craniofacial complex, particularly the mouth, is most consistently dysmorphic (Green et al. 1989; Lohr and Flynn 1993; O'Callaghan et al. 1991b), with anomalies of the hand being evident also, to suggest a process that may extend up to the middle of the second trimester (Bracha et al. 1991). Minor physical anomalies have been evaluated routinely with the Waldrop scale, an instrument that is subjective in application and insensitive to the range of anomalies actually encountered in practice; application of our newly developed scale for the detailed, quantitative assessment of such anomalies, based on anthropometric considerations (Lane et al. 1997), has elaborated particularly an excess of craniofacial dysmorphogenesis, primarily increased palatal height among overall narrowing and elongation of the middle and lower face, in schizophrenia. During this critical period in development, craniofacial morphogenesis follows a clear timeline, such that, for example, palatal morphology originates at 6–7 weeks and achieves postnatal form by 16–17 weeks of gestation (Cohen et al. 1993); head circumference at birth, which appears reduced in babies (particularly females and those without a family history of the disorder) who go on to manifest schizophrenia in early adulthood (McNeil et al. 1993), also appears to have identifiable antecedents by the 18th week (Barker et al. 1993).

Craniofacial development and cerebral structure development are so intimately related that not only might dysmorphogenesis in the former affect morphogenesis in the latter, but brain dysmorphogenesis would be expected to affect the developing mid-craniofacial region (Diewert and Wang 1992; Diewert et al. 1993). In our own MRI study, minor physical anomalies in schizophrenia appeared to be associated with poor premorbid intellectual function, particularly in females, and with a greater number of negative but not positive symptoms, particularly in males; such anomalies did not demonstrate any relationship to ventricular volume or to enlargement of cortical sulci but appeared to excess among those patients who evidenced qualitative developmental anomalies of cerebral structure that encompassed the ventricular system (O'Callaghan et al. 1995a).

Minor physical anomalies are held to have either (perhaps to a greater extent) genetic or (perhaps to a lesser extent) other, environmental origins (Smith 1988). The identification of "schizophrenia-like" psychosis in patients with genetically determined congenital disorders that include craniofacial dysmorphogenesis (e.g., Treacher Collins syndrome, as yet chromosomally unassigned [Nimgaonkar et al. 1993]; velocardiofacial syndrome, associated with deletions in the region of chromosome 22q11 [Pulver et al. 1994], which also appears to map a gene that is expressed during early embryogenesis [Halford et al. 1993]) is provocative; however, there is some dysmorphic overlap with a variety of other genetically determined developmental syndromes, such as Down syndrome, in which psychosis is not particularly common. Regarding palatal height, which particularly distinguishes schizophrenic patients from control subjects, there is a strong genetic component to variation therein (but not in palatal width or length), whereas it is palatal width and length (but not height) that are abnormal in Down syndrome (Shapiro 1969; Shapiro et al. 1967).

Most of those obstetric complications reported to occur to excess in schizophrenia concern the later phases of pregnancy and/or delivery and are thus unlikely candidates to "cause" phenomena having considerably earlier origins. However, in two independent studies (O'Callaghan et al. 1991b, 1995a), we have found bleeding in early pregnancy, the one complication reliably reported to occur considerably earlier in the course of pregnancy, to be associated particularly with the presence of anomalies in adult patients with schizophrenia. (It should be noted that a relationship between bleeding in early pregnancy and congenital anomalies in preterm offspring of low birthweight has been noted generally [Ornoy et al. 1976; Sipila et al. 1992]; such bleeding need not indicate a cause-and-effect relationship, but rather could reflect the failure of the uterus to follow through on the threat to expel a conceptus with preexisting malformation [O'Callaghan et al. 1991b].) It should be emphasized that bleeding in early pregnancy, preterm delivery and low birthweight, and minor physical anomalies appear to constitute a nexus of highly interrelated and sequential adversities (Crichton et al. 1972; Ornoy et al. 1976; Sipila et al. 1992); thus, the findings in schizophrenia would be further consistent with subtle dysfunction in a developmental process of early but otherwise uncertain origin that might both give rise to and interact with later, perinatal epiphenomena.

Cerebral Anomalies

As a potential counterpart of minor physical anomalies, a number of CT and MRI studies have indicated an excess in schizophrenia of structural brain anomalies of presumed neurodevelopmental origin. These can take the form of unexpectedly elevated (albeit still modest) rates of heterogeneous findings read as neurodevelopmental anomalies on blind qualitative evaluation of images (Scott et al. 1993; Waddington et al. 1990a) or excesses of individual anomalies.

Complete or partial agenesis of the corpus callosum (S. W. Lewis et al. 1988; Scott et al. 1993; Swayze et al. 1990; Waddington et al. 1990a), although rare, appears to occur at a heightened rate in schizophrenia; in the neuroradiological literature such callosal agenesis is an important indicator of other—particularly limbic developmental—anomalies of brain structure and appears to reflect dysgenesis occurring between the 6th–8th and the 18th–20th weeks of gestation (Atlas et al. 1986; Barkovich and Norman 1988). Cavum septum pellucidum also appears to excess in patients with schizophrenia (Degreef et al. 1992b; DeLisi et al. 1993; Jurjus et al. 1993; S. W. Lewis and Mezey 1985; Scott et al. 1993). Formation of the septum pellucidum is intimately related to the formation of other midline structures of the brain, particularly the corpus callosum (Schaefer et al. 1994), and the cavum anomaly of the septum pellucidum may carry similar implications regarding the timing of dysgenesis.

The Sylvian fissure/planum temporale region of the temporal lobe is known to be one of the most asymmetric in the human brain as the result of the evolution of (usually) left-hemisphere dominance for language function, and such asymmetry is disturbed in neurodevelopmental disorders such as dyslexia, autism, and learning disability. Evidence from recent MRI studies on the extent to which this "normal" asymmetry may be disturbed (DeLisi et al. 1994; Rossi et al. 1994) or remains intact (Bartley et al. 1993; Kleinschmidt et al. 1994) in schizophrenia is thus far inconsistent. Sylvian fissure asymmetry is normally evident in the fetal brain by the fourth month of pregnancy (Waddington 1993a), so those abnormalities observed would be in keeping with a close relationship between schizophrenia and disruption in the early development of (left) temporal lobe asymmetry (Crow et al. 1989).

Neuropathology and Neurochemistry

A new generation of neuropathological studies has emerged over the past decade and has contributed fundamentally to contemporary perspectives of schizophrenia. Some of these studies have suggested that schizophrenic patients show slight reductions in brain weight and length and in cerebral hemispheric and cortical volumes, as a putative counterpart to MRI studies (see first paragraph of this chapter). More consistently, such studies indicate increased ventricular size and highlight abnormalities in the temporal lobe—in particular, reduced volume of medial temporal lobe structures, such as the hippocampus and parahippocampal gyrus (entorhinal cortex)—and loss of Sylvian fissure asymmetry. There may also be reduced volume of the mediodorsal thalamus and abnormalities in pallidal/striatal structures and in the corpus callosum. In the hippocampus, parahippocampal gyrus, and cingulate and prefrontal cortices in particular, abnormalities have the patina not of neurodegenerative changes but rather of cytoarchitectonic anomalies that reflect disrupted neuronal migration during early to midgestation. Any disease that causes neuronal inflammation or degeneration in or beyond the last trimester will also cause proliferation of glial cells; the absence of gliosis in those regions showing cytoarchitectonic anomalies is an additional feature consistent with such an early origin (Akbarian et al. 1993a, 1993b; Benes 1993; Bogerts 1993; Waddington 1993a, 1993b).

At the neurochemical level, postmortem studies have revealed abnormalities in schizophrenic brains that are either consistent with or suggestive of an early, neurodevelopmental origin (Waddington 1993a, 1993b). In particular, the entorhinal cortex and subiculum of the hippocampal formation appear to show a selective reduction in the expression of two microtubule-associated proteins (MAP2 and MAP5) that contribute to the establishment and maintenance of local neuronal geometry in the absence of neuronal loss, gliosis, or other neurodegenerative markers (Arnold et al. 1991); reduced expression may be accompanied by selective reduction in hippocampal levels of synapsin I, a synaptic vesicle–associated phosphoprotein, in the absence of evidence for more general neuronal loss (Browning et al. 1993). Furthermore, both serum levels of neuron-specific enolase (Egan et al. 1992) and prefrontal levels of ubiquitination (Horton et al. 1993), two neurochemical markers of neurodegenerative processes, appear unaltered and are thus consistent with an early, neurodevelopmental origin for structural and cytoarchitectonic abnormalities of the brain in schizophrenia.

Neurodevelopmental Origins and Disease "Progression" in Schizophrenia

Onset of Psychosis: An Interaction With Normal Developmental and Maturational Processes?

If schizophrenia has its origins in disturbance(s) of fetal neurodevelopment that disrupt(s) the establishment of critical aspects of cerebral structure and function, perhaps including sexual dimorphism (Waddington 1993a), there remains the fundamental question of why the disease should stay "silent" for two or more decades before the emergence of psychotic symptoms. At one level, it can be argued that the disorder does *not* remain silent, but in fact manifests the sometimes subtle neuromotor and psychosocial deficits of infancy and childhood (see section above titled "A 'Readback' Analysis of Schizophrenia"), reflecting the impaired functioning of a brain already compromised in the earliest phase(s) of development. Yet it is still necessary to account for why these deficits do not typically include psychosis until the late teens or twenties. The most widely entertained explanation is that during the first two decades of life the brain is too immature to express the underlying neuronal abnormality in such a manner; it is not until the aberrant functional topography of the brain is codified, at the subsequent maturation of other associated systems or processes in critical brain regions, that "full blown" psychosis can be manifested (Murray and Lewis 1987; Waddington 1993a, 1993b; Walker 1994; Weinberger 1987).

Candidate systems and processes to determine delayed onset are numerous and not necessarily mutually exclusive. For example, cerebral function in the developing nervous system is influenced critically by the state of neuronal myelination, which can proceed at varying rates in differing regions of the brain. There is evidence that the prefrontal cortex completes myelination rather later than do other brain regions, and this evidence suggests some temporal contiguity with the emergence of psychosis in schizophrenia; however, although a somewhat similar time scale of adolescent myelination appears evident in the hippocampal region, the increased rate of hippocampal myelination in females would be inconsistent with their generally later onset of psychosis (Benes et al. 1994; Weinberger 1987). Synaptic pruning is a mechanism by which supernumerary and misdirected neurons that commonly arise in early neurodevelopment are progressively culled postnatally to allow competent functioning in the adult central nervous system. Thus, some temporal contiguity between such pruning and the emergence of psychosis in schizophrenia could reflect attainment in late adolescence of the functional maturity necessary to express psychosis; however, it should not be overlooked that hyper- (or, theoretically, hypo-) pruning could constitute a later, more direct pathophysiological mechanism by which psychosis is "generated" rather than "released" (Keshavan et al. 1994).

At least in nonhuman primates, dopaminergic and other monoaminergic innervations of the parahippocampal gyrus demonstrate a remarkably early appearance to complement that structure's precocious cytoarchitectonic differentiation during the first half of gestation (Berger et al. 1993; Kostovic et al. 1993), and might therefore be dysfunctional by way of temporal congruence with the cytoarchitectonic anomalies evident within this brain region in schizophrenia (see subsection above titled "Neuropathology and Neurochemistry"); likewise, dopaminergic innervation of the prefrontal cortex reaches its peak in late adolescence (Rosenberg and Lewis 1994), in some temporal congruence with the emergence of psychosis. In attempts to integrate variants of the classical dopamine hypothesis with a neurodevelopmental perspective, it has been argued that mesolimbic dopaminergic *hyper*function might represent a secondary, positive symptom–generating effect of negative symptom–generating dopaminergic *hypo*function in the frontal lobe, which is itself a consequence of developmentally determined temporal lobe abnormality (Davis et al. 1991; Jaskiw and Weinberger 1992). Finally, given that adolescence coincides with the attainment of maturity in a variety of neuroendocrine processes that have marked effects on brain function, including the modulation of dopaminergic systems, it has been argued that hormonal mechanisms may play a role in the emergence of psychosis, particularly in the context of gender differences in age at onset (Riecher-Rossler et al. 1994). It should not be overlooked that other, external events such as cerebral trauma (Buckley et al. 1993) can also precipitate the onset of psychosis in adulthood.

Chronic Illness: Static Encephalopathy Versus Disease Progression?

Following the onset of psychotic symptoms in schizophrenia, for whatever reason, a second fundamental and equally contentious question presents itself: is there an active disease process associated with "progression" over the chronic phase of the illness (DeLisi and Lieberman 1991; Waddington 1993b) during which very-long-term follow-up studies suggest heterogeneity in course and outcome (Waddington et al. 1995b)? Given that a variety of structural and functional abnormalities appear to be already present at the first psychotic episode (see section above titled "A 'Readback' Analysis of Schizophrenia"), one might begin by simply asking whether these abnormalities increase in magnitude over subsequent years of illness.

In brain-imaging studies, CT has been repeated over several years both in patients with early illness and in those with chronic illness (Vita et al. 1994; Waddington 1993b); however, the durations of such follow-up studies are modest. The problems of pseudo-longitudinal interpretation of MRI data from cross-sectional studies in chronically ill patients are considerable (Gur et al. 1994; O'Callaghan et al. 1992a); conversely, the most powerful approach to the issue—that is, prospective studies in first-episode patients—is still in its early stages (DeLisi et al. 1992). Although these various approaches have more commonly (albeit with some exceptions) failed to reveal evidence for prominently progressive increases in structural brain pathology, more detailed studies in larger numbers of patients over longer time frames are needed to resolve the matter; fortunately, such investigations are now in progress.

It has been argued, on the basis both of short-duration prospective and of less powerful cross-sectional studies, that cognitive dysfunction fails to show further deterioration beyond the period following the onset of psychosis and thus manifests the characteristics of a "static encephalopathy" (Goldberg et al. 1993; Heaton et al. 1994; Hyde et al. 1994). Conversely, on the basis of other cross-sectional studies, it has been argued that progressive cognitive deterioration ensues in the long term (Bilder et al. 1992). Indeed, the often-prominent cognitive deficits of some older, chronically ill patients continue to attract considerable attention (Buhrich et al. 1988; Goldberg et al. 1988; Purohit et al. 1993); these deficits can sometimes be so severe as to seem incompatible with an origin solely at or soon after the onset of psychosis in the absence of subsequent deterioration but do not appear to occur in association with postmortem neurochemical or neuropathological evidence of degenerative changes such as are found in dementia of the Alzheimer or other type (Casanova et al. 1993; El-Mallakh et al. 1991; Haroutunian et al. 1994; Purohit et al. 1993).

In our own prospective study among middle-aged, chronically ill inpatients already showing marked cognitive dysfunction at initial assessment, there was no overall deterioration 5 years later, while at 10 years there was a modest but significant deterioration that was essentially confined to males. However, the only patients to show prominent cognitive deterioration over the 10-year period were those evidencing the de novo emergence of tardive dyskinesia; those either consistently free of or persistently manifesting involuntary movements showed no such deterioration (Waddington and Youssef 1996a; Waddington et al. 1990b). New cases of tardive dyskinesia, even those manifesting late in the course of illness, appear to represent a special instance of marked cognitive (and other) deterioration that may be limited to the general period over which the involuntary movements emerge (Waddington 1995; Waddington et al. 1990b, 1993).

At the symptomatological level there exists perhaps more extensive (although still incomplete) evidence for some functional deterioration, particularly in terms of progression in negative symptoms over the first several years of illness (McGlashan and Fenton 1993). That the event most temporally congruent to progression in negative symptoms is the onset of positive psychotic symptoms may appear paradoxical. However, there is an emerging body of evidence to indicate that active psychosis, particularly when unchecked by neuroleptic drugs, may constitute an active morbid process associated with poorer long-term outcome in terms of extent of response to and relapse following such medication (Loebel et al. 1992; McEvoy et al. 1991; Wyatt 1991). In our own studies among a population of older, chronically ill inpatients, many of whom had been admitted in the preneuroleptic era, increasing duration of initially untreated psychosis was associated (after controlling for the patient's age and the duration and continuity of subsequent neuroleptic treatment) with increasing prominence of negative symptoms and cognitive dysfunction (Scully et al. 1997; Waddington et al. 1995b). Negative symptoms continue to show associations with poor premorbid function and can be present early in the course of illness, where they serve as an adverse prognosticand (Andreasen et al. 1990; Kelley et al. 1992; McGlashan and Fenton 1992). Thus, our data suggest that the pathophysiology underlying active, unchecked psychosis may be associated with further progression of these features. However, the biological basis of such a process remains obscure.

Although a "static encephalopathy" appears more readily compatible with contemporary perspectives of schizophrenia as a neurodevelopmental disorder, it must be emphasized that some "progressive" element to schizophrenia would not in itself contradict such a perspective; early, neurodevelopmental origin and later, adult disease progression are not mutually exclusive and may be sequential phases of one longitudinal process or separate dimensions of the same pathology. The emergence of psychosis may reflect the triggering of an active morbid process that, particularly when unchecked by antipsychotic drugs, constitutes one element in a sequence of events that link neurodevelopmental disturbance to the progressive determination of outcome in the long term (Waddington et al. 1998).

Integration and Speculation: A "Cascade" Process?

As previously noted, the long-standing battle lines between proponents of the "genetic" versus the "environmental" origins of schizophrenia are manned by increasingly entrenched troops; a genetic component to schizophrenia appears both well-established and strong, with environmental factors often posited to represent an alternative or else an additive source of risk within a classical multifactorial–polygenic threshold model of liability for the disorder (Waddington 1993a). However, it is not clear that risk factors must be either "genetic" *or* "environmental" in any exclusive sense. For example, in Down syndrome, a neurodevelopmental disorder of genetic/chromosomal origin, the totality of maldevelopment evident may be influenced in part by maternal exposure to environmental factors (Khoury and Erickson 1992; Shapiro 1994); the abnormal genotype, although causal for the disorder, may result in a lack of protective buffering against deleterious environmental factors that might be mediated, at least in part, via altered immunological function (Nespoli et al. 1993). Furthermore, the neurodevelopmental origins of Down syndrome are associated not with a "static encephalopathy" but rather with precocious progression to neurodegenerative brain changes in later life (Jorgensen et al. 1990; Mann et al. 1990). Similarly, it may be that the gene(s) predisposing to schizophrenia both code for dysgenesis and confer on individuals some varying epigenetic susceptibility to other prenatally dysgenic factors (Waddington 1993a). Fluctuating asymmetry (random differences in size, in either direction, between supposedly identical right- and left-sided structures) is a putative index of developmental stability—that is, an organism's capacity to develop as determined genetically despite adverse environmental conditions; dermatoglyphic examination suggests that such developmental stability may be compromised in schizophrenia in a manner consistent with early or midgestational dysmorphogenesis (Markow 1992; Mellor 1992).

Furthermore, the primary (genetic?) factor(s) that determine why an *individual* develops a given disorder may not be the same factors that determine why so many in a *population* of individuals develop that same condition; an environmental factor that is common may, by increasing everyone's risk by a very small amount, result in many more individuals crossing some threshold of risk for the condition, although it would be difficult to pinpoint any one individual whose illness had been specifically "caused" by that factor (Khaw 1994). At a more speculative level, it has been argued that for dysmorphic disorders showing non-Mendelian patterns of inheritance, *randomness* is inherent in morphogenesis; furthermore, a *stochastic* (probabilistic) single-gene model can generate continuous liability curves very similar to those postulated by multifactorial–polygenic threshold models (Kurnit et al. 1987). With the entry of schizophrenia to the ranks of dysmorphic disorders, such theorizing assumes a new relevance for the continuing debate on these issues (Waddington 1993a, 1994).

Conclusion

In overview, one might speculate that schizophrenia should be viewed in terms of a "cascade" process: intrauterine events (genetically misprogrammed or environmentally determined) appear to disrupt the establishment of fundamental aspects of brain structure and function; these intrauterine events are associated with the evolution of sometimes subtle neuromotor and psychosocial abnormalities over the course of subsequent development during infancy and childhood; psychosis is typically released in late adolescence or early adulthood only when this abnormal functional topography of the brain is codified on completion of maturation in other associated systems or processes; release of psychosis reflects the triggering of an active morbid process that, particularly when unchecked by or unresponsive to antipsychotic medication, results in the clinical deterioration that can be particularly evident over those years immediately following the first psychotic episode; later in life, deterioration (or, sometimes, clinical amelioration) may reflect the additional impact of the heterogeneous processes of human aging. It should not be overlooked that the consequences of such later processes on a brain compromised early in neurodevelopment may differ from their impact on an otherwise "normal" brain.

There remain many fundamental questions concerning not only the nature and timing of dysmorphic events in schizophrenia but also the process(es) by which these events might result in the evolution of symptoms and the overall course of illness; also, the extent to which such concepts apply also to affective psychosis (Van Os et al. 1995) requires further study. It is perhaps unlikely that a single causative agent and disease process can account for all cases of schizophrenia, but how homogeneous or otherwise is the disorder? Given the diversity of early intrauterine adversity, what specific factor(s) determine differentiation into schizophrenia rather than into other, more classical neurodevelopmental disorders? Such notions of schizophrenia as a disease of very early origin but with an evolving pathophysiology and course determined by the sequential interplay of developmental, maturational, and aging processes may repay further exploration. More specific elucidation of the nature of neurodevelopmental disturbances that might lead to the coming "on stream" of an active disease process only in adulthood, as reflected in unchecked psychotic symptoms (Waddington et al. 1998), could hold fundamental clues to the basis of the disorder.

References

Akbarian S, Bunney WE, Potkin SG, et al: Altered distribution of nicotinamide–adenine dinucleotide phosphate–diaphorase cells in frontal lobe of schizophrenics implies disturbances of cortical development. Arch Gen Psychiatry 50:169–177, 1993a

Akbarian S, Vinuela A, Kim JJ, et al: Distorted distribution of nicotinamide–adenine dinucleotide phosphate–diaphorase neurons in temporal lobe of schizophrenics implies anomalous cortical development. Arch Gen Psychiatry 50:178–187, 1993b

Andreasen NC, Flaum M, Swayze VW, et al: Positive and negative symptoms in schizophrenia. Arch Gen Psychiatry 47:615–621, 1990

Andreasen NC, Rezai K, Alliger R, et al: Hypofrontality in neuroleptic-naive patients and in patients with chronic schizophrenia. Arch Gen Psychiatry 49:943–958, 1992

Andreasen NC, Arndt S, Swayze V, et al: Thalamic abnormalities in schizophrenia visualized through magnetic resonance image averaging. Science 266:294–298, 1994

Arnold SE, Lee VM-Y, Gur RE, et al: Abnormal expression of two microtubule-associated proteins (MAP2 and MAP5) in specific subfields of the hippocampal formation in schizophrenia. Proc Natl Acad Sci U S A 88:10850–10854, 1991

Atlas SW, Zimmerman RA, Bilaniuk LT, et al: Corpus callosum and limbic system: neuroanatomic MR evaluation of developmental anomalies. Radiology 160:355–362, 1986

Barker DJP, Osmond C, Simmonds SJ, et al: The relation of small head circumference and thinness at birth to death from cardiovascular disease in adult life. BMJ 306:422–426, 1993

Barkovich AJ, Norman D: Anomalies of the corpus callosum: correlation with further anomalies of the brain. AJNR Am J Neuroradiol 9:493–501, 1988

Bartley AJ, Jones DW, Torrey EF, et al: Sylvian fissure asymmetries in monozygotic twins: a test of laterality in schizophrenia. Biol Psychiatry 34:853–863, 1993

Benes FM: Neurobiological investigations in cingulate cortex of schizophrenic brain. Schizophr Bull 19:537–549, 1993

Benes FM, Turtle M, Khan Y, et al: Myelination of a key relay zone in the hippocampal formation occurs in the human brain during childhood, adolescence, and adulthood. Arch Gen Psychiatry 51:477–484, 1994

Berger B, Alvarez C, Goldman-Rakic PS: Neurochemical development of the hippocampal region in the fetal rhesus monkey, I: early appearance of peptides, calcium-binding proteins, DARPP-32, and monoamine innervation in the entorhinal cortex during the first half of gestation (E47 to E90). Hippocampus 3:279–305, 1993

Bilder RM, Lipschutz-Broch L, Reiter G, et al: Intellectual deficits in first-episode schizophrenia: evidence for progressive deterioration. Schizophr Bull 18:437–448, 1992

Blanchard JJ, Neale JM: The neuropsychological signature of schizophrenia: generalized or differential deficit? Am J Psychiatry 151:40–48, 1994

Bogerts B: Recent advances in the neuropathology of schizophrenia. Schizophr Bull 19:431–445, 1993

Bogerts B, Ashtari M, Degreef G, et al: Reduced temporal limbic structure volumes on magnetic resonance images in first-episode schizophrenia. Psychiatry Res 35:1–13, 1990

Bracha HS, Torrey EF, Bigelow LB, et al: Subtle signs of prenatal maldevelopment of the hand ectoderm in schizophrenia: a preliminary monozygotic twin study. Biol Psychiatry 30:719–725, 1991

Bradbury TN, Miller GA: Season of birth in schizophrenia: a review of evidence, methodology, and etiology. Psychol Bull 98:569–594, 1985

Browning MD, Dudek EM, Rapier JL, et al: Significant reductions in synapsin but not synaptophysin specific activity in the brains of some schizophrenics. Biol Psychiatry 34:529–535, 1993

Buchsbaum MS, Haier RJ, Potkin SG, et al: Frontostriatal disorder of cerebral metabolism in never-medicated schizophrenics. Arch Gen Psychiatry 49:935–942, 1992

Buckley P, Stack JP, Madigan C, et al: Magnetic resonance imaging of schizophrenia-like psychoses associated with cerebral trauma: clinico-pathological correlates. Am J Psychiatry 150:146–148, 1993

Buhrich N, Crow TJ, Johnstone EC, et al: Age disorientation in chronic schizophrenia is not associated with premorbid intellectual impairment or past physical treatment. Br J Psychiatry 152:466–469, 1988

Buka SL, Tsuang MT, Lipsitt LP: Pregnancy/delivery complications and psychiatric diagnosis. Arch Gen Psychiatry 50:151–156, 1993

Cannon TD, Mednick SA, Parnas J, et al: Developmental brain abnormalities in the offspring of schizophrenic mothers, I: contributions of genetic and perinatal factors. Arch Gen Psychiatry 50:551–564, 1993

Carpenter WT Jr, Buchanan RW: Schizophrenia. N Engl J Med 330:681–690, 1994

Casanova MF, Carosella NW, Gold JM, et al: A topographical study of senile plaques and neurofibrillary tangles in the hippocampi of patients with Alzheimer's disease and cognitively impaired patients with schizophrenia. Psychiatry Res 49:41–62, 1993

Chamberlain G: Vaginal bleeding in early pregnancy—I. BMJ 302:1141–1143, 1991

Cohen SR, Chen L, Trotman CA, et al: Soft-palate myogenesis: a developmental field paradigm. Cleft Palate Craniofac J 30:441–446, 1993

Cooper DW, Brennecke SP, Wilton AN: Genetics of pre-eclampsia. Hypertension in Pregnancy 12:1–23, 1993

Crichton JU, Dunn HG, McBurney AK, et al: Minor congenital defects in children of low birth weight. J Pediatr 80:830–832, 1972

Crow TJ, Ball J, Bloom SR, et al: Schizophrenia as an anomaly of development of cerebral asymmetry. Arch Gen Psychiatry 46:1145–1150, 1989

Davis KL, Kahn RS, Ko G, et al: Dopamine in schizophrenia: a review and reconceptualization. Am J Psychiatry 148:1474–1486, 1991

Degreef G, Ashtari M, Bogerts B, et al: Volumes of ventricular system subdivisions measured from magnetic resonance images in first-episode schizophrenic patients. Arch Gen Psychiatry 49:531–537, 1992a

Degreef G, Bogerts B, Falkai P, et al: Increased prevalence of the cavum septum pellucidum in magnetic resonance scans and post-mortem brains of schizophrenic patients. Psychiatry Res 45:1–13, 1992b

DeLisi LE, Lieberman JA: Longitudinal perspectives on the pathophysiology of schizophrenia: examining the neurodevelopmental vs neurodegenerative hypotheses. Schizophr Res 5:183–210, 1991

DeLisi LE, Hoff AL, Schwartz JE, et al: Brain morphology in first episode schizophrenia-like psychotic patients: a quantitative magnetic resonance imaging study. Biol Psychiatry 29:159–175, 1991

DeLisi LE, Stritzke P, Riordan H, et al: The timing of brain morphological changes in schizophrenia and their relationship to clinical outcome. Biol Psychiatry 31:241–254, 1992

DeLisi LE, Hoff AL, Kushner M, et al: Increased prevalence of cavum septum pellucidum in schizophrenia. Psychiatry Res 50:193–199, 1993

DeLisi LE, Hoff AL, Neale C, et al: Asymmetries in the superior temporal lobe in male and female first-episode schizophrenic patients: measures of the planum temporale and superior temporal gyrus by MRI. Schizophr Res 12:19–28, 1994

Diewert VM, Wang KY: Recent advances in primary palate and midface morphogenesis research. Crit Rev Oral Biol Med 4:111–130, 1992

Diewert VM, Lozanoff S, Choy V: Computer reconstructions of human embryonic craniofacial morphology showing changes in relations between the face and brain during primary palate formation. J Craniofac Genet Dev Biol 13:184–192, 1993

Done DJ, Johnstone EC, Frith CD, et al: Complications of pregnancy and delivery in relation to psychosis in adult life: data from the British perinatal mortality survey sample. BMJ 302:1576–1580, 1991

Done DJ, Crow TJ, Johnstone EC, et al: Childhood antecedents of schizophrenia and affective illness: social adjustment at ages 7 and 11. BMJ 309:699–703, 1994

Eagles JM: Is schizophrenia disappearing? Br J Psychiatry 158:834–835, 1991

Eagles JM, Gibson J, Bremner MH, et al: Obstetric complications in DSM-III schizophrenics and their siblings. Lancet 336:1139–1141, 1990

Egan MF, El-Mallakh RS, Suddath RL, et al: Cerebrospinal fluid and serum levels of neuron-specific enolase in patients with schizophrenia. Psychiatry Res 43:187–195, 1992

El-Mallakh RS, Kirch DG, Shelton R, et al: The nucleus basalis of Meynert, senile plaques, and intellectual impairment in schizophrenia. J Neuropsychiatry Clin Neurosci 3:383–386, 1991

Fish B, Marcus J, Hans SL, et al: Infants at risk for schizophrenia: sequelae of a genetic neurointegrative defect. Arch Gen Psychiatry 49:221–235, 1992

Geddes JR, Lawrie SM: Obstetric complications and schizophrenia: a meta-analysis. Br J Psychiatry 167:786–793, 1995

Gillberg C: Do children with autism have March birthdays? Acta Psychiatr Scand 82:152–156, 1990

Goldberg TE, Kleinman JE, Daniel DG, et al: Dementia praecox revisited: age disorientation, mental status and ventricular enlargement. Br J Psychiatry 153:187–190, 1988

Goldberg TE, Hyde TM, Kleinman JE, et al: Course of schizophrenia: neuropsychological evidence for a static encephalopathy. Schizophr Bull 19:797–804, 1993

Green MF, Satz P, Gaier DJ, et al: Minor physical anomalies in schizophrenia. Schizophr Bull 15:91–99, 1989

Gunther-Genta F, Bovet P, Hohlfeld P: Obstetric complications and schizophrenia: a case–control study. Br J Psychiatry 164:165–170, 1994

Gur RE, Pearlson GD: Neuroimaging in schizophrenia research. Schizophr Bull 19:337–353, 1993

Gur RE, Mozley PD, Shtasel DL, et al: Clinical subtypes of schizophrenia: differences in brain and CSF volume. Am J Psychiatry 151:343–350, 1994

Hafner H, Haas S, Pfeifer-Kurda M, et al: Abnormal seasonality of schizophrenia births. European Archives of Psychiatry and Neurological Sciences 236:333–342, 1987

Halford S, Wilson DI, Daw SCM, et al: Isolation of a gene expressed during early embryogenesis from the region of 22q11 commonly deleted in DiGeorge syndrome. Hum Mol Genet 2:1577–1583, 1993

Haroutunian V, Davidson M, Kanof PD, et al: Cortical cholinergic markers in schizophrenia. Schizophr Res 12:137–144, 1994

Harvey I, Ron MA, Du Boulay G, et al: Reduction of cortical volume in schizophrenia on magnetic resonance imaging. Psychol Med 23:591–604, 1993

Heaton R, Paulsen JS, McAdams LA, et al: Neuropsychological deficits in schizophrenics. Arch Gen Psychiatry 51:469–476, 1994

Heun R, Maier W: The role of obstetric complications in schizophrenia. J Nerv Ment Dis 181:220–226, 1993

Hoff AL, Riordan H, O'Donnell DW, et al: Neuropsychological functioning in first-episode schizophreniform patients. Am J Psychiatry 149: 898–903, 1992

Horton K, Forsythe CS, Sibtain N, et al: Ubiquitination as a probe for neurodegeneration in the brain in schizophrenia: the prefrontal cortex. Psychiatry Res 48:145–152, 1993

Hyde TM, Nawroz S, Goldberg TE, et al: Is there cognitive decline in schizophrenia? a cross-sectional study. Br J Psychiatry 164:494–500, 1994

Jaskiw GE, Weinberger DR: Dopamine and schizophrenia: a cortically correct perspective. Seminars in the Neurosciences 4:179–188, 1992

Jones P, Rodgers B, Murray R, et al: Child developmental risk factors for adult schizophrenia in the British 1946 birth cohort. Lancet 344: 1398–1402, 1994

Jones PB, Rantakallio P, Hartikainen AL, et al: Schizophrenia as a long-term outcome of pregnancy, delivery, and perinatal complications: a 28-year follow-up of the 1966 north Finland general population birth cohort. Am J Psychiatry 155:355–364, 1998

Jorgensen OS, Brooksbank BW, Balazs R: Neuronal plasticity and astrocytic reaction in Down syndrome and Alzheimer disease. J Neurol Sci 98:63–79, 1990

Jurjus GJ, Nasrallah HA, Olson SC, et al: Cavum septum pellucidum in schizophrenia, affective disorder and healthy controls: a magnetic resonance imaging study. Psychol Med 23:319–322, 1993

Kelley ME, Gilbertson M, Mouton A, et al: Deterioration in premorbid functioning in schizophrenia: a developmental model of negative symptoms in drug-free patients. Am J Psychiatry 149:1543–1548, 1992

Kendell RE, Adams W: Unexplained fluctuations in the risk for schizophrenia by month and year of birth. Br J Psychiatry 158:758–763, 1991

Kendell RE, Kemp IW: Winter-born versus summer-born schizophrenics. Br J Psychiatry 151:499–505, 1987

Keshavan M, Anderson S, Pettegrew JW: Is schizophrenia due to excessive synaptic pruning in the prefrontal cortex? The Feinberg hypothesis revisited. J Psychiatr Res 28:239–265, 1994

Khaw KT: Genetics and environment: Geoffrey Rowe revisited. Lancet 343:838–839, 1994

Khoury MJ, Erickson JD: Can maternal risk factors influence the presence of major birth defects in infants with Down syndrome? Am J Med Genet 43:1016–1022, 1992

Kleinschmidt A, Falkai P, Huang Y, et al: In vivo morphometry of planum temporale asymmetry in first-episode schizophrenia. Schizophr Res 12:9–18, 1994

Kostovic I, Petanjek Z, Judas M: Early areal differentiation of the human cerebral cortex: entorhinal area. Hippocampus 3:447–458, 1993

Kurnit DM, Layton WM, Matthysse S: Genetics, chance and morphogenesis. Am J Hum Genet 41:979–995, 1987

Kwon JS, Shenton ME, Hirayasu Y, et al: MRI study of cavum septi pellucidi in schizophrenia, affective disorder, and schizotypal personality disorder. Am J Psychiatry 155:509–515, 1998

Lane A, Kinsell A, Murphy P, et al: The anthropometric assessment of dysmorphic features in schizophrenia as an index of its developmental origins. Psychol Med 27:1155–1164, 1997

Lewis G, David A, Andreasson S, et al: Schizophrenia and city life. Lancet 340:137–140, 1992

Lewis MS: Age incidence and schizophrenia, I: the season of birth controversy. Schizophr Bull 15:59–73, 1989

Lewis SW, Mezey CC: Clinical correlates of septum pellucidum cavities: an unusual association with psychosis. Psychol Med 15:43–54, 1985

Lewis SW, Murray RM: Obstetric complications, neurodevelopmental deviance, and risk of schizophrenia. J Psychiatr Res 21:413–421, 1987

Lewis SW, Reveley MA, David AS, et al: Agenesis of the corpus callosum and schizophrenia: a case report. Psychol Med 18:341–347, 1988

Livingston R, Adam BS, Bracha HS: Season of birth and neurodevelopmental disorders: summer birth is associated with dyslexia. J Am Acad Child Adolesc Psychiatry 32:612–616, 1993

Loebel AD, Lieberman JA, Alvir JMJ, et al: Duration of psychosis and outcome in first-episode schizophrenia. Am J Psychiatry 149:1183–1188, 1992

Lohr JB, Flynn K: Minor physical anomalies in schizophrenia and mood disorders. Schizophr Bull 19:551–556, 1993

Mann DMA, Royston MC, Ravindra CR: Some morphometric observations on the brains of patients with Down's syndrome: their relationship to age and dementia. J Neurol Sci 99:154–164, 1990

Markow TA: Genetics and developmental stability: an integrative conjecture on aetiology and neurobiology of schizophrenia. Psychol Med 22:295–305, 1992

McCreadie RG, Hall DJ, Berry IJ, et al: The Nithsdale schizophrenia surveys X: obstetric complications, family history and abnormal movements. Br J Psychiatry 161:799–805, 1992

McEvoy JP, Schooler NR, Wilson WH: Predictors of therapeutic response to haloperidol in acute schizophrenia. Psychopharmacol Bull 27:97–101, 1991

McGlashan TH, Fenton WS: The positive-negative distinction in schizophrenia. Arch Gen Psychiatry 49:63–72, 1992

McGlashan TH, Fenton WS: Subtype progression and pathophysiologic deterioration in early schizophrenia. Schizophr Bull 19:71–84, 1993

McNeil TF: Obstetric complications in schizophrenic parents. Schizophr Res 5:89–101, 1991

McNeil TF, Cantor-Graae E, Nordstrom LG, et al: Head circumference in "preschizophrenic" and control neonates. Br J Psychiatry 162:517–523, 1993

Mellor CS: Dermatoglyphic evidence of fluctuating asymmetry in schizophrenia. Br J Psychiatry 160:467–472, 1992

Murray RM, Lewis SW: Is schizophrenia a neurodevelopmental disorder? BMJ 295:681–682, 1987

Nespoli L, Burgio GR, Ugazio AG, et al: Immunological features of Down's syndrome: a review. J Intellect Disabil Res 37:543–551, 1993

Nimgaonkar VL, Scott JA, Brar JS, et al: Co-occurrence of schizophrenia and Treacher Collins syndrome. Am J Med Genet 48:156–158, 1993

O'Callaghan E, Larkin C, Kinsella A, et al: Obstetric complications, the putative familial sporadic distinction, and tardive dyskinesia in schizophrenia. Br J Psychiatry 157:578–584, 1990

O'Callaghan E, Gibson T, Colohan HA, et al: Season of birth in schizophrenia: evidence for confinement of an excess of winter births to patients without a family history of mental disorder. Br J Psychiatry 158:764–769, 1991a

O'Callaghan E, Larkin C, Kinsella A, et al: Familial, obstetric, and other clinical correlates of minor physical anomalies in schizophrenia. Am J Psychiatry 148:479–483, 1991b

O'Callaghan E, Buckley P, Redmond O, et al: Abnormalities of cerebral structure in schizophrenia on magnetic resonance imaging: interpretation in relation to the neurodevelopmental hypothesis. J R Soc Med 85:227–231, 1992a

O'Callaghan E, Gibson T, Colohan HA, et al: Risk of schizophrenia in adults born after obstetric complications and their association with early onset of illness: a controlled study. BMJ 305:1256–1259, 1992b

O'Callaghan E, Buckley P, Madigan C, et al: The relationship of minor physical anomalies and other putative indices of neurodevelopmental disturbance in schizophrenia to abnormalities of cerebral structure on MRI. Biol Psychiatry 38:516–524, 1995a

O'Callaghan E, Cotter D, Colgan C, et al: Confinement of winter birth excess in schizophrenia to the urban-born and its gender specificity. Br J Psychiatry 166:51–54, 1995b

Ohlund LS, Ohman A, Alm T, et al: Season of birth and electrodermal unresponsiveness in male schizophrenics. Biol Psychiatry 27:328–340, 1990

Ornoy A, Benady S, Kohen-Raz R, et al: Association between maternal bleeding during gestation and congenital anomalies in the offspring. Am J Obstet Gynecol 124:474–478, 1976

Pallast EG, Jongbloet PH, Straatman HM, et al: Excess seasonality of births among patients with schizophrenia and seasonal ovopathy. Schizophr Bull 20:269–276, 1994

Pettegrew JA, Keshaven MS, Panchalingam K, et al: Alterations in brain high-energy phosphate and membrane phospholipid metabolism in first-episode, drug-naive schizophrenics. Arch Gen Psychiatry 48: 563–568, 1991

Pulver AE, Liang KY, Brown CH, et al: Risk factors for schizophrenia: season of birth, gender, and familial risk. Br J Psychiatry 160:65–71, 1992

Pulver AE, Nestadt G, Goldberg R, et al: Psychotic illness in patients diagnosed with velo-cardio-facial syndrome and their relatives. J Nerv Ment Dis 182:476–478, 1994

Purohit DP, Davidson M, Perl DP, et al: Severe cognitive impairment in elderly schizophrenic patients: a clinicopathological study. Biol Psychiatry 33:255–260, 1993

Reading R, Raybould S, Jarvis S: Deprivation, low birth weight, and children's height: a comparison between rural and urban areas. BMJ 307: 1458–1462, 1993

Riecher-Rossler A, Hafner H, Dutsch-Strobel A, et al: Further evidence for a specific role of estradiol in schizophrenia? Biol Psychiatry 36:492–494, 1994

Rosenberg DR, Lewis DA: Changes in the dopaminergic innervation of monkey prefrontal cortex during late postnatal development: a tyrosine hydroxylase immunohistochemical study. Biol Psychiatry 36:272–277, 1994

Rossi A, Serio A, Stratta P, et al: Planum temporale asymmetry and thought disorder in schizophrenia. Schizophr Res 12:1–7, 1994

Rubin P, Karle A, Moller-Madsen S, et al: Computerised tomography in newly diagnosed schizophrenia and schizophreniform disorder. Br J Psychiatry 163:604–612, 1993

Rubin P, Homl S, Madsen PL, et al: Regional cerebral blood flow distributed in newly diagnosed schizophrenia and schizophreniform disorder. Psychiatry Res 53:57–75, 1994

Russell D, Douglas AS, Allan TM: Changing seasonality of birth—a possible environmental effect. J Epidemiol Community Health 47:362–367, 1993

Sacchetti E, Calzeroni A, Vita A, et al: The brain damage hypothesis of the seasonality of births in schizophrenia and major affective disorders: evidence from computerized tomography. Br J Psychiatry 160:390–397, 1992

Sanders RD, Keskavan MS, Schooler NR: Neurological examination abnormalities in neuroleptic-naive patients with first-break schizophrenia: preliminary results. Am J Psychiatry 151:1231–1233, 1994

Sartorius N, Jablenski A, Korten G, et al: Early manifestations and first-contact incidence of schizophrenia in different cultures: a preliminary report on the initial evaluation of the WHO Collaborative Study on determinants of outcome of severe mental disorders. Psychol Med 16:909–928, 1986

Saykin AJ, Shtasel DL, Gur RE, et al: Neuropsychological deficits in neuroleptic naive patients with first-episode schizophrenia. Arch Gen Psychiatry 51:124–131, 1994

Schaefer GB, Bodensteiner JB, Thompson JN: Subtle anomalies of the septum pellucidum and neurodevelopmental deficits. Dev Med Child Neurol 36:554–559, 1994

Schlaepfer TE, Harris GJ, Tien AY, et al: Decreased regional cortical gray matter volume in schizophrenia. Am J Psychiatry 151:842–848, 1994

Schroder J, Niethammer R, Geider FJ, et al: Neurological soft signs in schizophrenia. Schizophr Res 6:25–30, 1992

Scott TF, Price TRP, George MS, et al: Midline cerebral malformations and schizophrenia. J Neuropsychiatry Clin Neurosci 5:287–293, 1993

Scully PJ, Coakley G, Kinsella A, et al: Psychopathology, executive (frontal) and general cognitive impairment in relation to duration of initially untreated versus subsequently treated psychosis in chronic schizophrenia. Psychol Med 27:1303–1310, 1997

Shapiro BL: A twin study of palatal dimensions partitioning genetic and environmental contributions to variability. Angle Orthod 39:139–151, 1969

Shapiro BL: The environmental basis of the Down syndrome phenotype. Dev Med Child Neurol 36:84–90, 1994

Shapiro BL, Gorlin RJ, Redman RS, et al: The palate and Down's syndrome. N Engl J Med 276:1460–1463, 1967

Sipila P, Hartikainen-Sorri AL, Oja H, et al: Perinatal outcome of pregnancies complicated by vaginal bleeding. Br J Obstet Gynaecol 99:959–963, 1992

Sival DA: Studies on fetal motor behavior in normal and complicated pregnancies. Early Hum Dev 34:13–20, 1993

Smith DW: Recognizable Patterns of Human Malformation. Philadelphia, PA, WB Saunders, 1988

Swayze VW, Andreasen NC, Ehrhardt YC, et al: Developmental abnormalities of the corpus callosum in schizophrenia. Arch Neurol 47:805–808, 1990

Torrey EF: Prevalence studies in schizophrenia. Br J Psychiatry 150:598–608, 1987

Torrey EF, Bowler AE, Watson CG, et al: The seasonality of schizophrenic births: a reply to Marc S. Lewis. Schizophr Bull 16:1–15, 1990

Torrey EF, Bowler AE, Rawlings R, et al: Seasonality of schizophrenia and stillbirths. Schizophr Bull 19:557–562, 1993

Van Os J, Jones P, Lewis G, et al: Developmental precursors of affective illness in a general population birth cohort. Arch Gen Psychiatry 54:625–631, 1995

Verdoux H, Bourgeois M: A comparative study of obstetric history in schizophrenia, bipolar patients and normal subjects. Schizophr Res 9:67–69, 1993

Vita A, Giobbio GM, Dieci M, et al: Stability of cerebral ventricular size from the appearance of the first psychotic symptoms to the later diagnosis of schizophrenia. Biol Psychiatry 35:960–962, 1994

Waddington JL: Schizophrenia: developmental neuroscience and pathobiology. Lancet 341:531–536, 1993a

Waddington JL: Neurodynamics of abnormalities in cerebral metabolism and structure in schizophrenia. Schizophr Bull 19:55–69, 1993b

Waddington JL: Genetics, chance and dysmorphogenesis in schizophrenia. Br J Psychiatry 165:693–694, 1994

Waddington JL: Psychological and cognitive correlates of tardive dyskinesia in schizophrenia and other disorders treated with neuroleptic drugs, in Behavioral Neurology of Movement Disorders. Edited by Weiner WJ, Long AE. New York, Raven, 1995, pp 43–53

Waddington JL, Youssef HA: Evidence for a gender-specific decline in the rate of schizophrenia in rural Ireland over a 50-year period. Br J Psychiatry 164:171–176, 1994

Waddington JL, Youssef HA: Cognitive dysfunction in schizophrenia followed prospectively over 10 years and its longitudinal relationship to the emergence of tardive dyskinesia. Psychol Med 26:681–688, 1996a

Waddington JL, Youssef HA: Familial-genetic and reproductive epidemiology of schizophrenia in rural Ireland: age at onset, familial morbid risk and parental fertility. Acta Psychiatr Scand 93:62–68, 1996b

Waddington JL, O'Callaghan E, Larkin C, et al: Magnetic resonance imaging and spectroscopy in schizophrenia. Br J Psychiatry 157 (suppl 9): 56–65, 1990a

Waddington JL, Youssef HA, Kinsella A: Cognitive dysfunction in schizophrenia followed up over 5 years, and its longitudinal relationship to the emergence of tardive dyskinesia. Psychol Med 20:835–842, 1990b

Waddington JL, O'Callaghan E, Larkin C, et al: Cognitive dysfunction in schizophrenia: organic vulnerability factor or state marker for tardive dyskinesia? Brain Cogn 23:56–70, 1993

Waddington JL, O'Callaghan E, Youssef HA, et al: The neurodevelopmental basis to schizophrenia: beyond a hypothesis, in Schizophrenia—An Integrated View. Edited by Fog R, Gerlach J, Hemmingsen P, et al. Copenhagen, Denmark, Munksgaard, 1995a, pp 43–53

Waddington JL, Youssef HA, Kinsella A: Sequential cross-sectional and 10-year prospective study of severe negative symptoms in relation to duration of initially untreated psychosis in chronic schizophrenia. Psychol Med 25:849–857, 1995b

Waddington JL, Lane A, Scully PJ, et al: Neurodevelopmental and neuro-progressive processes in schizophrenia. Psychiatr Clin North Am 21: 123–149, 1998

Walker EF: Developmentally moderated expressions of the neuropathology underlying schizophrenia. Schizophr Bull 20:453–480, 1994

Walker EF, Savoie T, Davis D: Neuromotor precursors of schizophrenia. Schizophr Bull 20:441–451, 1994

Weinberger DR: Implications of normal brain development for the pathogenesis of schizophrenia. Arch Gen Psychiatry 44:660–669, 1987

Williams MA, Mittendorf R, Lieberman E, et al: Adverse infant outcomes associated with first-trimester vaginal bleeding. Obstet Gynecol 78:14–18, 1991

Wyatt RJ: Neuroleptics and the natural course of schizophrenia. Schizophr Bull 17:325–351, 1991

Youssef HA, Kinsella A, Waddington JL: Evidence for geographical variations in the prevalence of schizophrenia in rural Ireland. Arch Gen Psychiatry 48:254–258, 1991

Youssef HA, Kinsella A, Waddington JL: Gender specificity of geographical variations in morbid risk for schizophrenia in rural Ireland. Acta Psychiatr Scand 88:135–139, 1993

Zipursky RB, Marsh L, Lim KO, et al: Volumetric MRI assessment of temporal lobe structures in schizophrenia. Biol Psychiatry 35:501–516, 1994

Chapter 2

Interaction of Genes and Prenatal Exposures in Schizophrenia

Dolores Malaspina, M.D., Nancy L. Sohler, M.P.H., and
Ezra S. Susser, M.D., Dr.P.H.

From the outset of schizophrenia research it was recognized that the relatives of patients were often "tainted by hereditary mental disease" (Bleuler 1911). It was also apparent that genetic vulnerability alone might not account for schizophrenia. Thus, it has long been acknowledged that an understanding of both genetic and environmental factors may be necessary to explain the complexities of the illness.

Nonetheless, research on the interaction of genetic and prenatal factors in schizophrenia did not develop until recently. While significant advances were made in early research on both genetic and prenatal exposures in schizophrenia, these studies were rarely designed to examine the interaction of these exposures. By *interaction*, we mean not only that both genes and prenatal exposures are related to the disease but also that prenatal exposures modify the expression of genes (and vice versa).

Research on gene–environment interaction has now begun dramatic growth. The breakthrough can be attributed to the emergence of a conceptual framework and of well-defined research strategies, as well as to new technologies. In this chapter we introduce the reader to this developing field of research in schizophrenia, describing in turn 1) genetic epidemiological research that strongly suggests some sort of multifactorial causation of schizophrenia; 2) some basic models of multifactorial causation, which can include both genetic and environmental factors; 3) current evidence for gene–environment interaction in schizophrenia; and 4) new research designed to investigate interactions between genes and prenatal exposures in schizophrenia.

Genetic Epidemiological Studies of Schizophrenia

Studies that attempt to isolate the effects of genes from those of the environment in disease causation, and that consider the interplay of genes and environment, fall within the sphere of *genetic epidemiology*. During the past decade, genetic epidemiologists have identified specific genetic causes for several neuropsychiatric illnesses. In most cases, these disorders are transmitted in a simple Mendelian fashion, such as occurs in Huntington's disease or myotonic dystrophy.

In contrast to these disorders, which follow simple inheritance patterns, schizophrenia and many other neuropsychiatric disorders have a complex pattern of familial transmission and an unknown mode of inheritance. Several phenomena may be responsible for this complexity: *incomplete penetrance*, wherein additional environmental factors may be necessary for the genetic causes to be expressed as manifest disorder; *epistasis*, where the disorder may result from the interaction of several major genes; *variable expressivity*, in which a single genetic form of the disorder may have several phenotypic expressions (e.g., some nonschizophrenic psychiatric diagnoses in the family may represent alternative expressions of a gene); *diagnostic instability*, such that a subject's diagnostic status may change over time; and *etiological heterogeneity*, under which an ordinarily genetic syndrome may have sporadic (environmentally produced) forms, known as "phenocopies," as well as a variety of genetic forms resulting from disruption in a number of different genes, a condition known as "nonallelic" heterogeneity.

This degree of complexity poses special problems for studies that seek to differentiate genetic from nongenetic causes. Genetic causation of a complex disorder can range from a point mutation in single genes to polygenic causes that entail epistasis (genetic interaction) among the several genes involved. Healthy individuals in the pedigree may yet carry some genetic predisposition for schizophrenia. A classical linkage analysis is difficult to sustain in the face of such complexity in gene expression.

Perhaps because of these difficulties, genetic epidemiologists have not succeeded in identifying specific genes that cause schizophrenia. Indeed, the search for genetic linkage in schizophrenia has often been frustrating, although several potential gene linkages have been identified (for example, see Kalsi et al. 1995 and Schizophrenia Collaborative Linkage Group 1996 [linkages to 22q11–q13]; Antonarakis et al. 1995, Gurling et al. 1995, Mowry et al. 1995, and Kaufman et al. 1998 [linkages to 6p23]; and Farone et al. 1998 and Straub et al. 1998 [linkages to 10p]).

Yet this failure to "find the gene" should not obscure the major results that have emerged from research examining the genetic epidemiology of schizophrenia and the fundamental implications of these results for the etiologies of the disease (Susser and Susser 1992). Taken together, these results suggest that the genetic risk for schizophrenia entails several genes rather than a single gene; that genes often confer a vulnerability to the disease that has a variable expression, depending on other genetic or environmental exposures; and that genes are not the only cause of schizophrenia. In this section we summarize these findings and discuss the implications for etiology.

Genetic Risk Entails Several Genes

Results from genetic epidemiological research suggest that a single gene is unlikely to cause schizophrenia (Cloninger 1994; Kringlen 1993; Parnas et al. 1982; Prescott and Gottesman 1993; Stabenau and Pollin 1993). In genetic modeling of pedigree data, the sharp drop in risk observed as one moves from monozygotic twins to siblings and offspring, and then to second- and third-degree relatives, is more than can be explained under a monogenic model. Thus, the results of genetic modeling studies strongly suggest some sort of multifactorial causation—either multiple genes or genes plus environmental factors.

An oligogenic model, which involves several genes rather than one gene, was initially proposed by Karlsson (1972), who suggested a two-locus hypothesis for the inheritance of schizophrenia. Oligogenic models can explain the sharp drop in risk with genetic distance described above. These models also can account for the increased familial recurrence rates that are observed in relatives of more severely affected probands (Gottesman and Shields 1982; Odegaard 1972).

Genes Confer a Vulnerability

Genetic epidemiological studies have consistently found that what is inherited by many individuals is a vulnerability to schizophrenia rather than the disorder itself. Indeed, the evidence suggests that the phenotype known as schizophrenia may represent only the severe end of a spectrum of phenotypes that can result from a genetic predisposition. This variation in gene expression may have several outcomes: no psychiatric illness, schizophrenia-spectrum disorders, individual symptoms (such as social anxiety) (Torgersen et al. 1993), or even other psychiatric diagnoses (Farmer et al. 1987; Gershon et al. 1988; Maier et al. 1993, Rosenthal 1970). These genes may also confer subtle differences in neuropsychological or neurophysiological functioning on nonpsychiatrically ill family members (Holzman 1992; Levy et al. 1994).

Of these possible outcomes, schizophrenia-spectrum disorders represent perhaps the best-known manifestation of "schizophrenia vulnerability genes." This family of disorders may contain several types of other nonaffective psychoses, including schizoaffective disorder, schizotypal personality disorder, paranoid personality disorder, and perhaps other atypical psychoses. The frequency of some or all of these disorders is consistently found to be increased among the biological relatives of schizophrenic probands (Baron et al. 1981, 1983; Kendler and Gruenberg 1984; Kendler et al. 1985, 1994; Kety et al. 1975, 1994).

The fact that purported schizophrenia vulnerability genes may have such different phenotypic expressions strongly suggests that additional etiological factors must be involved. One possibility is that schizophrenia vulnerability genes might interact with other genes via epistasis. A second possibility is that schizophrenia vulnerability genes may interact with prenatal exposure or another environmental factor in disease causation. Of course, these two possibilities are not mutually exclusive.

Genes Are Not the Only Cause

Using classical strategies of genetic epidemiology such as twin and adoption studies, researchers have firmly established the importance of genes in the causation of schizophrenia. These investigations have also suggested, however, that environmental etiologies may be similarly important. Thus, in twin studies, if fully penetrant genes alone accounted for the illness, then the monozygotic (MZ) concordances should be close to 100% rather than the 40%–70% observed (Gottesman and Shields 1982). A twin study by Suddath and colleagues (1990) of MZ twin pairs discordant for schizophrenia yielded still more compelling evidence for the role of environment. Among these twin pairs, brain abnormalities associated with schizophrenia, such as increased ventricular size and diminished volume of temporolimbic structures, were almost always more prominent in the affected than in the unaffected co-twin. Because MZ twins share 100% of their genetic material, these differences between affected and unaffected co-twins can be presumed to be epigenetic in origin. In this case, the epigenetic factor was likely to be a prenatal or perinatal environmental factor; in utero brain insult is a well-documented environmental cause of ventricular enlargement.

Implications for Etiology

The findings described above suggest that the risk of schizophrenia can be influenced by multiple genes and also by prenatal or other environmental exposures. What, then, is the relationship between these causes—and, in particular, between the genetic causes, on the one hand, and the environmental causes, on the other?

The simplest view is that either genes—albeit multiple genes—or environment can be sufficient to cause the illness, and that the majority of cases are either primarily genetic or primarily environmental in origin. This is the model adopted in studies that attempt to reduce heterogeneity by dividing schizophrenia into familial and sporadic subtypes. This is also the model implicit in genetic studies that consider environmentally induced cases as "phenocopies" (also termed "sporadics," i.e., genetically nonsusceptible but nonetheless affected individuals). This simple model is not easily reconciled, however, with the findings described previously. Since genetic vulnerability may manifest as various diseases or as no disease, genetic vulnerability alone is often not sufficient to cause schizophrenia.

A view that is more compatible with the data is that of multifactorial causation. In its most general form, this view holds that many factors confer an increased risk for a disease but these factors are not related to the disease in a one-to-one manner. In most cases, the disease results from the combined action of several risk factors. Multifactorial causation is thought to apply to a broad range of chronic diseases, including myocardial infarction, diabetes, and some neurodevelopmental disorders.

Multifactorial causation does not, however, represent a single model of causation; rather, it encompasses several distinct models, each of which has been found to apply for some diseases. In the following section we describe basic models of multifactorial causation, which can include both genetic and environmental factors.

Models of Multifactorial Causation

Although there are many ways in which genes and prenatal exposures can combine to produce schizophrenia, there is still no consensus as to the most useful conceptual framework for categorizing these processes. Here we will adhere to a framework that emerged through a synthesis of concepts from the fields of epidemiology and genetics (Ottman 1996; Susser and Susser 1992).

Basic Models of Multifactorial Causation

Below we describe three generally accepted models of multi-factorial causation, as well as a fourth model that is commonly adopted but controversial. Our descriptions apply to circumstances in which genetic and environmental factors *increase* the risk of disease. It is important to note that the same models can be applied to circumstances in which these factors are *protective* against diseases. Also, other, more complex circumstances can often be subsumed by an elaboration of these models.

Models such as those we describe are useful in genetic epidemiology for testing hypotheses about the ways several risk factors combine to cause disease (see Darroch 1997). Each model predicts certain patterns in observed genetic epidemiological data; the model can be ruled out if the data are not compatible with the prediction. At the same time, a given pattern of observed data can be compatible with more than one model, so that one cannot always determine the underlying nature of the multifactorial causation from the data.

Additive-Effects Model

Under an additive-effects model that includes both a genetic and an environmental risk factor, the effect of one factor does not depend on the effect of the other. The combined effect of both factors on the risk of disease is simply the sum of their individual effects, after accounting for "parallelism" (Darroch 1997). Parallelism arises because individuals who have *both* risk factors could get the disease from *either* factor. Thus, the two risk factors "compete" to cause the disease. Under the additive-effects model, the combined effect of two risk factors is less than the sum of their individual effects in populations where parallelism exists.

To illustrate an additive effect, let us assume that the lifetime risk of schizophrenia is influenced by a specific gene and by a specific prenatal exposure. Assume that the risk of schizophrenia in individuals with neither the gene nor the prenatal exposure is 0.005. Now assume that the lifetime risk of schizophrenia in individuals with the gene (only) is increased by 0.010—that is, from 0.005 to 0.015—and that the prenatal exposure increases the risk by the same amount. Under the additive-effects model, the lifetime risk of schizophrenia in individuals with both risk factors would be increased at most by 0.010 + 0.010 = 0.020, resulting in a lifetime risk of 0.005 + 0.020 = 0.025. (The actual lifetime risk would be less than 0.025, depending on the amount of parallelism that exists in the population.)

An additive-effects model may apply when the relevant genetic and environmental risk factors act at the same point in the causal path; that is, if they are alternate means to the same end. For example, a genetic defect or a prenatal insult may disrupt neuronal migration during early gestation. Disrupted neuronal migration—regardless of its cause—may then increase the risk of schizophrenia.

Synergistic-Effects Model

Genetic and environmental risk factors are synergistic if they interact biologically to cause disease. This implies that some individuals could not get the disease from exposure to *either* the genetic or the environmental factors, but could get the disease from exposure to *both* factors. Thus, under the synergistic-effects model, the combined effect of both factors on the risk of disease is generally expected to be greater than the sum of the individual effects of each factor.

To illustrate this scenario, again assume that the lifetime risk of schizophrenia is influenced by a specific gene and a specific prenatal exposure and that the risk in individuals with neither the gene nor the prenatal exposure is 0.005. Now consider that the gene causes the disease in the presence of the prenatal exposure, but does not cause the disease in the absence of the prenatal exposure. Among individuals with both the gene and the prenatal exposure, the disease risk could be dramatically increased. Among individuals with only the gene, however, the risk of disease would remain 0.005.

Biological synergy among risk factors is common in nature. Insulin-dependent diabetes mellitus provides an illustration of this phenomenon (Solimena and DeCamilli 1995): some cases of insulin-dependent diabetes mellitus may result from a human leukocyte antigen haplotype that is expressed as a disease after the occurrence of an autoimmune response to Coxsackie virus infection.

Neural tube defects (NTDs) such as spina bifida and anencephaly provide an example of biological synergism in neurodevelopmental disorders. Studies suggest that fetal NTDs may be caused by a genetic defect in homocysteine metabolism when maternal intake of folate in early gestation is low (Mills et al. 1995; van der Put et al. 1995). The genetic defect impedes the metabolism of homocysteine, whereas folate has the opposite effect. Therefore, if folate intake in early gestation is high, the effect of the genetic defect on the risk of an NTD in the fetus may be minimal. On the other hand, if folate intake in early gestation is low, the genetic defect may confer a high risk of an NTD in the fetus.

Mediating-Effects Model

Under a mediating-effects model, it is assumed that a genetic risk factor does not directly influence the risk of schizophrenia. Rather, the gene influences the chance of exposure to environmental factor(s), which in turn influences the risk of schizophrenia. An example of this model would be a situation in which a gene is associated with an increased risk of sustaining head trauma, and head trauma increases the risk of developing schizophrenia. In this case, the gene is not thought to cause schizophrenia directly, but rather to influence the risk of disease through a third factor, head trauma.

Examples of mediating effects in schizophrenia can include prenatal exposures as well. Consider that a maternal gene may confer susceptibility to influenza, including to maternal influenza during pregnancy. In utero exposure to influenza may increase the risk of schizophrenia in the offspring. In this example, the maternal gene influences the risk of schizophrenia in offspring by increasing the risk of prenatal exposure to influenza.

Similarly, the effects of environmental factors on schizophrenia can be mediated by genes. An environmental exposure might turn on or turn off a gene that increases the risk of schizophrenia (Bloom 1993; Kandel 1998).

Multiplicative-Effects Model

Some contend that a multiplicative-effects model represents another way that genetic and environmental risk factors can relate to each other in schizophrenia. Under the multiplicative-effects model, the combined effect of a genetic and environmental risk factor is the product of their independent effects. For instance, if the odds ratio for a genetic risk factor is 3, and the odds ratio for a prenatal exposure is also 3, the odds of schizophrenia in individuals with both risk factors is expected to be 9 times greater than that in individuals with neither risk factor.

Others argue that when factors that influence the risk of disease follow a multiplicative-effects model, they are acting synergistically and should be considered a special case of the synergistic-effects model (Darroch 1997; Koopman 1981; Rothman and Greenland 1998). A example of this is a circumstance in which disease is thought to be caused in two stages. A genetic factor is associated with the risk of the first stage of disease but not the second stage. An environmental factor is associated with the risk of the second stage of disease but not the first. The first stage can occur without manifesting itself as disease unless it is followed by the second stage; conversely, the second stage will not cause disease unless it is preceded by the first stage. Provided that the occurrence of each stage is independent of the other, the risk of disease in this example is the product of the risks associated with each of the (genetic and environmental) factors. This is a special case of the synergistic model because both the first stage and the second stage are required for the disease; thus, *both* the genetic factor and the environmental factor must be present to produce disease.

Nonetheless, multiplicative effects are implicit in many statistical analyses of genetic and epidemiologic data and in study designs to explore the relationship between genetic and environmental risk factors (e.g., "case-only" study, as described in Khoury and Flanders 1996). Hence, it may still be useful to consider the multiplicative-effects model separately.

Ecumenical Viewpoint

Viewed from an ecumenical perspective, the models described above are not mutually exclusive; rather, they coexist. Each model applies only to some cases of the disease.

In schizophrenia, it is highly unlikely that any one of these models applies to all or even to most cases. It is more likely that multiple genes, and multiple environmental exposures, can affect the risk of the disease, and that these are capable of combining in many different ways to produce the disease. Thus, the ecumenical viewpoint seems most appropriate. This argument has been made forcefully by Gottesman (1991), who coined the term *ecumenical* to refer to a circumstance in which a variety of models play a role in some cases.

Gene–Environment Interaction

The concept of interaction between causes evolved separately in the fields of genetics and epidemiology and is not fully developed in either field. Some geneticists include all of the models described above under the concept of interaction. Epidemiologists, on the other hand, are more restrictive in defining interaction; for them, interaction between risk factors occurs when the effect of one factor is dependent on the presence of another. This can occur in several ways, two of which were described in the previous section: parallelism, in which two factors present in the same individual "compete" to cause disease, and biological synergy, in which two factors act synergistically to cause disease, such that an individual will get the disease when exposed to both risk factors but not when exposed to either alone.

In the remainder of this chapter we focus on biological synergy between genes and prenatal factors. However, we will continue to use the more familiar term "gene–environment interaction," with the caveat that we are referring to synergy rather than parallelism.

Evidence for Gene–Environment Interaction

For schizophrenia, the investigation of models of multifactorial causation is still in its infancy. The evidence obtained thus far does suggest, however, that many cases of schizophrenia involve inter-actions between genetic and environmental causes, as reviewed below. Evidence supporting the occurrence of gene–environment interaction can be found in published results of family, twin, adop-tion, and high-risk studies.

Family Studies

Today, virtually no one disputes that schizophrenia runs in some families. Familial aggregation of this disease has been demon-strated in a large body of research dating back to the 19th century (Rudin 1916; Kallman 1946; Gottesman and Shields 1982 [review]). Diseases that run in families may, however, be multifactorial in ori-gin and may entail both genetic and environmental causation to varying degrees. These causes may or may not exhibit interaction as previously defined.

Family History and Season of Birth

Several family studies have suggested an interaction between winter–spring season of birth and genetic vulnerability to schizophrenia. Some of these studies compared family history of schizophrenia in patients born during the winter or spring (December to May) with that in patients born in the summer or autumn (June to November) and found that patients born in the winter or spring were more likely to have a family history (Lo 1985; Owens and Lewis 1988). Pulver and colleagues (1992) compared schizophrenic patients born in different months with regard to the morbid risk for schizo-phrenia before age 30 years among first-degree relatives. Among probands born in February through May, the risk of schizophrenia among first-degree relatives was dramatically increased.

This finding has not been consistent across all studies. A few studies actually suggest that patients born during the winter and spring are *less* likely to have a family history of schizophrenia (Kinney and Jakobsen 1978; O'Callaghan et al. 1991; Shur 1982). Nonetheless, the preponderance of the evidence indicates that fac-tors associated with season of birth may interact with genetic vul-nerability to cause schizophrenia.

Family History and Country of Birth

A family history approach was used by Sugarman and Craufurd (1994) in an attempt to explain the high rates of schizophrenia observed among the Afro-Caribbean population in Britain. The authors found that Afro-Caribbean–born parents of probands with schizophrenia had recurrence rates similar to those of British-born control subjects, but that British-born siblings of the probands had increased rates of schizophrenia. Sugarman and Craufurd surmised that these findings could be due to an interaction between a genetic vulnerability present in this ethnic group and exposure to an environmental factor in Britain, such as prenatal rubella infection (Glover 1989) or cannabis use (Andreasson et al. 1987).

Family History and Obstetric Complications

Some family studies suggest that environmental factors may interact with genetic predisposition to influence the phenotypic expression of schizophrenia, even if the psychiatric illness arises independent of the environmental factor. For example, Stober and colleagues (1993) found that among individuals with a family history of schizophrenia, rates of exposure to obstetric complications were similar in schizophrenic patients and control subjects; yet patients exposed to obstetric complications had significantly earlier hospitalizations than did those unexposed to such complications.

Twin Studies

As is well known, twin studies represent an effective means of isolating the genetic contribution to a disease. MZ and dizygotic (DZ) twin pairs share 100% and 50% of their genes, respectively, and may share the same familial environment. Thus, when genetic factors are important in a disorder's etiology, the MZ and DZ co-twins of probands should differ in their risk for the disorder. As a result, the comparison of concordance rates for MZ and DZ twins can give compelling evidence of genetic causation in schizophrenia. As reviewed by Kendler (1986), MZ and DZ co-twins of probands with schizophrenia differ in their risk for the disorder, with weighted mean probandwise concordances of approximately 59% and 15%, respectively.

Twin studies are often used to estimate a disorder's *heritability*, that is, the amount of variance explained by genetic factors as opposed to environmental factors (Cannon et al. 1998). However, heritability estimates are based on the assumption of no gene–environment interaction (Khoury et al. 1993; Schwartz 1998). They are also time and environment specific and dependent on the relative variation of genetic and environmental factors in the particular population under investigation. For example, the same genetic factor, distributed the same way within a population, may elicit different heritability estimates due solely to differences in the prevalence of the environmental factors (Plomin 1990).

The potential use of twin studies in the detection of gene–environment interaction is less widely appreciated. Yet twin studies have provided some of the most important data to support the occurrence of interaction. A landmark study by Fischer (1971) demonstrated that discordant MZ twins may have similar genetic loading for the disorder. In this follow-up study of the offspring of discordant MZ twins, the offspring of affected and unaffected co-twins had similarly increased rates of schizophrenia. A more recent study by Gottesman and Bertelsen (1989), which extended the time of follow-up of the Fischer sample, supported this observation (although a similar study by Kringlen [1987] did not). The parsimonious explanation for these findings is that an environmental exposure is required for the expression of the genotype or that an inhibitory environmental factor in the unaffected co-twin represses the genotype's expression.

More recently, differences in the neurological status of twin pairs have been used to shed light on gene–environment interaction. Davis and Phelps (1995) used handedness in MZ twin pairs as a marker of placentation status, defined as monochorionic (shared chorion) or dichorionic (separate chorions). They found higher concordance rates of schizophrenia in presumed monochorionic MZ twin pairs (60%) than in dichorionic pairs (32%), a finding consistent with the view that a shared prenatal exposure such as in utero infection was required to cause the disease.

Adoption Studies

Adoption studies represent another strategy for differentiating genetic from environmental effects. The adoptee method was initially used in schizophrenia in a study by Heston (1966). He found a significantly greater risk for schizophrenia among the adopted offspring of schizophrenic mothers than among the adopted offspring of control mothers. Later adoption studies replicated and extended this finding (Rosenthal et al. 1968; Tienari et al. 1983), supporting a strong genetic contribution to schizophrenia (Gottesman and Shields 1982; Kendler et al. 1994; Kety et al. 1994; Wender et al. 1974). Taken together, these adoption studies have convincingly demonstrated that the familial transmission of schizophrenia cannot be explained by familial transmission of the postnatal environment. It should be noted, however, that these studies do not rule out a contribution of the *prenatal* environment to familial transmission of schizophrenia; by definition, prenatal exposures occur before the offspring are separated from their biological mothers.

Adoption studies in Finland have extended the method to ascertain the role of both genes and environment in risk for schizophrenia (Tienari and Wynne 1994; Tienari et al. 1983, 1994). In addition to comparing rates of schizophrenia in adoptees with and without schizophrenic biological parents, the investigators also conducted assessments of adoptive families. The findings suggested that the genetic vulnerability to schizophrenia was expressed only in the presence of a disturbed family environment. Although these researchers did not examine prenatal exposures, their findings add further to the evidence that environmental factors may interact with genes to increase disease penetrance.

High-Risk Studies

High-risk studies generally follow children of schizophrenic patients; the parental condition marks the children as genetically at high risk for the disorder (Mednick and McNeil 1968). Approximately 10%–15% of so-called high-risk children become schizophrenic (Gottesman 1978). Under the *premise* of synergistic effects between genes and environmental factors, one can identify, in a high-risk cohort, environmental exposures that markedly increase risk and can therefore *infer* that such factors modify the genetic risk.

An interactive effect was implicated in a high-risk study by Cannon and colleagues (1993). The authors used "neither, one, or two parents with schizophrenia related disorders" to mark three categories of genetic vulnerability for schizophrenia. They then examined the contribution of obstetric complications to ventricular enlargement among individuals in each of these categories of genetic risk. The effect of obstetric complications on ventricular enlargement was greater among individuals at high genetic risk than among those at low genetic risk. Thus, genetic risk modified the effect of obstetric complications and vice versa.

In a second example of the high-risk strategy, Walker and colleagues (1981) used electrodermal responsiveness as a marker of genetic vulnerability in high-risk group members. They examined the association between paternal absence and risk of schizophrenia. Paternal absence had a significant effect only in the group that was defined as genetically vulnerable, a finding supportive of a gene–environment interaction.

Unfortunately, the potential of this method for the study of gene–environment interaction has not been fully realized. In most high-risk studies, statistical power was low and prenatal exposures were not precisely measured. The few studies that have been able to investigate interaction, however, have found evidence for it.

Summary

Although far from conclusive, the studies reviewed in this section suggest that some form of gene–environment interaction plays an important role in a portion of schizophrenia cases. Future research may take the further step of distinguishing between the models described in the previous section. The data that would be required to make these distinctions have been specified to some degree

(Kendler and Eaves 1986); however, currently available data are not sufficient for this purpose.

New Research

As previously noted, research to date has supported the presence of a gene–environment interaction in schizophrenia but has not allowed for any precise statements on the nature of this interaction. Chief among the limitations of this research were the reliance on imprecise data on both the genetic and environmental exposures and the inability to measure both exposures in the same individuals.

Genetic factors were often assessed only by family history in parents. In most studies, environmental factors were assessed by similarly imprecise methods. For instance, for prenatal exposure data, studies often used maternal recall or routine midwifery records.

Moreover, recent studies that have applied more rigorous methods to the assessment of either genetic or prenatal exposures have not included equally rigorous assessments of both exposures, as required to examine interaction. Genetic linkage studies were not able to collect data on prenatal exposures. Similarly, studies that examined prenatal exposures, such as those presented elsewhere in this volume, generally lacked precise genetic data.

Gene–Environment Interaction

Thus, methodological advances are needed to better elucidate gene–environment interactions in schizophrenia. These advances are within sight: ongoing studies are already applying new methods that offer the possibility of fundamental advances in this field. Our research team has undertaken two studies that illustrate some of the approaches being used.

The first is an extension of the Dutch Famine Study (see Chapter 6, this volume), which was based on the "natural experiment" of the Dutch Hunger Winter of 1944–1945. One hypothesis we are exploring is that low prenatal intake of folate may interact with a genetic defect to cause schizophrenia. The Dutch Hunger Winter struck at a precisely circumscribed time and place, and in a society able to document the timing and severity of the nutritional deprivation. The prenatal exposure was relatively homogenous across cohorts affected by the famine, making this study a powerful design for the detection of genetic factors that confer a vulnerability to developing schizophrenia after prenatal insult. Thus, we will test our hypothesis by comparing famine-exposed schizophrenia case subjects with unexposed case and control subjects with respect to the genetic defect.

The second study, Prenatal Determinants of Schizophrenia, is a population-based birth cohort investigation that was designed specifically to examine different kinds of prenatal exposures in schizophrenia (Susser et al., in press). One of the hypotheses we are testing is that the occurrence of maternal viral infection interacts with a genetic predisposition in the etiology of schizophrenia. Although previous research has suggested that prenatal exposure to maternal influenza and rubella infection, for example, may increase the risk of schizophrenia (see Chapter 5, this volume), these studies could not achieve precise measures of exposure and have yielded inconsistent results. In the Prenatal Determinants of Schizophrenia study, however, *prenatal* serum samples were drawn from the mothers of birth cohort members and were frozen and stored, providing us now with precise serologic measures of exposure to maternal viral infection. At the same time, family history data and blood samples drawn from cohort members as adults will provide us with precise data on genetic factors, ultimately allowing a rigorous test of the role of this gene–environment interaction in the etiology of schizophrenia.

Conclusion

Schizophrenia has a complex genetic picture that may be characterized by reduced penetrance, variable expressivity, and both genetic and nongenetic heterogeneity. We propose that elucidation of the genetics of this complex disorder will require investigations of both genetic and environmental mechanisms in disease causation. Thus, an understanding of the potential relationships between genes and prenatal exposures provides a necessary framework for understanding the process of disease pathogenesis. Even if prenatal or perinatal exposures contribute to only a minority of schizophrenia cases, such exposures may have a significant impact on individuals with a genetic vulnerability; genetic factors may be necessary but not sufficient for the development of illness.

To achieve this goal, we will need to apply emerging technology that has dramatically enhanced the precision of exposure data. The potential for increased precision applies not only for genetic but also for prenatal exposure data. Many of the required technologies are already available. It is critical that schizophrenia researchers recognize the necessity of research designs in which data on genetic and prenatal exposures are obtained within the same study and are combined in analyses that relate such exposure to schizophrenia risk.

References

Andreasson S, Allebeck P, Engstroem A, et al: Cannabis and schizophrenia: a longitudinal study of Swedish conscripts. Lancet 2:1483–1486, 1987

Antonarakis SE, Blouin JL, Pulver AE, et al: Schizophrenia susceptibility and chromosome 6p24–22 (letter). Nat Genet 11:235–236, 1995

Baron M, Asnis L, Gruen R: The Schedule for Schizotypal Personalities (SSP): a diagnostic interview for schizotypal features. Psychiatry Res 4:213–228, 1981

Baron M, Asnis L, Gruen R: Plasma amine oxidase and genetic vulnerability to schizophrenia. Arch Gen Psychiatry 40:275–279, 1983

Bleuler E: Dementia Praecox, or the Group of Schizophrenias. Leipzig, Deuticke, 1911

Bloom FE: Advancing a neurodevelopmental origin for schizophrenia. Arch Gen Psychiatry 50:224–227, 1993

Cannon TD, Mednick SA, Parnas J, et al: Developmental brain abnormalities in the offspring of schizophrenic mothers, I: contributions of genetic and perinatal factors. Arch Gen Psychiatry 50:551–564, 1993

Cannon TD, Kaprio J, Lonnqvist J, et al: The genetic epidemiology of schizophrenia in a Finnish twin cohort: a population-based modeling study. Arch Gen Psychiatry 55:67–74, 1998

Cloninger CR: Turning point in the design of linkage studies of schizophrenia. Am J Med Genet 15:54:83–92, 1994

Darroch D: Biologic synergism and parallelism. Am J Epidemiol 145: 661–668, 1997

Davis JO, Phelps JA: Twins with schizophrenia: genes or germs? Schizophr Bull 21:13–18, 1995

Farmer AE, McGuffin P, Gottesman II: Twin concordance for DSM-III schizophrenia: scrutinizing the validity of the definition. Arch Gen Psychiatry 44:634–641, 1987

Farone SV, Matise T, Svrakic D, et al: Genome scan of European-American schizophrenia pedigrees: results of the NIMH Genetics Initiated Millennium Schizophrenia Consortium. Am J Med Genet 81:290–295, 1998

Fischer M: Psychoses in the offspring of schizophrenic monozygotic twins and their normal co-twins. Br J Psychiatry 118:43–52, 1971

Gershon ES, DeLisi LE, Hamovit J, et al: A controlled family study of chronic psychosis. Arch Gen Psychiatry 45:328–336, 1988

Glover GR: Why is there a high rate of schizophrenia in British Caribbeans? Br J Hosp Med 42:48–51, 1989

Gottesman I: Schizophrenia and genetics: where are we? are you sure? in The Nature of Schizophrenia: New Approaches to Research and Treatment. Edited by Wynne L, Cromwell R, Matthysse S. New York, Wiley, 1978, pp 59–69

Gottesman II: Schizophrenia Genesis: The Origins of Madness. New York, Freeman, 1991

Gottesman II, Bertelsen A: Confirming unexpressed genotypes for schizophrenia: risks in the offspring of Fischer's Danish identical and fraternal discordant twins. Arch Gen Psychiatry 46:867–872, 1989

Gottesman II, Shields J: Schizophrenia: The Epigenetic Puzzle. Cambridge, England, Cambridge University Press, 1982

Gurling H, Kalsi G, Chen AH, et al: Schizophrenia susceptibility and chromosome 6p24–22. Nat Genet 11:234–235, 1995

Heston LL: Psychiatric disorders in foster home reared children of schizophrenic mothers. Br J Psychiatry 112:819–825, 1966

Holzman PS: Behavioral markers of schizophrenia useful for genetic studies. J Psychiatr Res 26:427–445, 1992

Kallman FJ: The genetic theory of schizophrenia. Am J Psychiatry 103: 309–322, 1946

Kalsi G, Brynjolfsson J, Butler R, et al: Linkage analysis of chromosome 22q12–13 in a United Kingdom/Icelandic sample of 23 multiplex schizophrenia families. Am J Med Genet 60:298–301, 1995

Kandel ER: A new intellectual framework for psychiatry. Am J Psychiatry 155:457–469, 1998

Karlsson JL: A two-locus hypothesis for inheritance of schizophrenia, in Genetic Factors in Schizophrenia. Edited by Kaplan AR. Springfield, IL, Charles C Thomas, 1972, pp 246–255

Kaufmann CA, Suarez B, Malaspina D, et al: NIMH Genetics Initiated Millennium Schizophrenia Consortium: linkage analysis of African-American pedigrees. Am J Med Genet 81:282–289, 1998

Kendler KS: Genetics of schizophrenia, in Psychiatry Update: The American Psychiatric Association Annual Review, Vol 5. Edited by Frances AJ, Hales RE. Washington, DC, American Psychiatric Press, 1986, pp 25–41

Kendler KS, Eaves LJ: Models for the joint effect of genotype and environment on liability to psychiatric illness. Am J Psychiatry 143:279–289, 1986

Kendler KS, Gruenberg AM: An independent analysis of the Copenhagen sample of the Danish adoption study, VI: the pattern of psychiatric illness, as defined by DSM-III in adoptees and relatives. Arch Gen Psychiatry 41:555–564, 1984

Kendler KS, Gruenberg AM, Tsuang MT: Psychiatric illness in first-degree relatives of schizophrenic and surgical control patients. Arch Gen Psychiatry 42:770–779, 1985

Kendler KS, Gruenberg AM, Kinney DK: Independent diagnoses of adoptees and relatives as defined by DSM-III in the provincial and national samples of the Danish Adoption Study of Schizophrenia. Arch Gen Psychiatry 51:456–468, 1994

Kety SS, Rosenthal D, Wender PH, et al: Mental illness in the biological and adoptive families of adopted individuals who have become schizophrenic: a preliminary report based on psychiatric interviews, in Genetic Research in Psychiatry. Edited by Fieve RR, Rosenthal D, Brill H. Baltimore, MD, Johns Hopkins University Press, 1975, pp 147–166

Kety SS, Wender PH, Jakobsen B, et al: Mental illness in the biological and adoptive relatives of schizophrenic adoptees: replication of the Copenhagen Study in the rest of Denmark. Arch Gen Psychiatry 51: 442–455, 1994

Khoury MJ, Flanders WD: Nontraditional approaches in the analysis of gene-environment interaction: case-control studies with no controls! Am J Epidemiology 144:207–213, 1996

Khoury M, Beaty T, Cohen B: Fundamentals of Genetic Epidemiology. New York, Oxford University Press, 1993

Kinney DF, Jakobsen B: Environmental factors in schizophrenia: new adoption study evidence, in The Nature of Schizophrenia: New Approaches to Research and Treatment. Edited by Wynne LW, Cromwell RL, Matthysse S. New York, Wiley, 1978, pp 38–51

Koopman JS: Interaction between discrete causes. Am J Epidemiol 113:716–724, 1981

Kringlen E: Contributions of genetic studies on schizophrenia, in Search for the Causes of Schizophrenia. Edited by Hafner H, Gattaz WF, Janzarik W. New York, Springer-Verlag, 1987, pp 123–143

Kringlen E: Genes and environment in mental illness: perspectives and ideas for future research. Acta Psychiatr Scand Suppl 370:79–84, 1993

Levy DL, Holzman PS, Matthysse S, et al: Eye tracking and schizophrenia. Schizophr Bull 20:47–62, 1994

Lo CW: Season of birth of schizophrenics in Hong Kong. Br J Psychiatry 147:212–213, 1985

Maier W, Lichterman D, Minges J, et al: Continuity and discontinuity of affective disorders and schizophrenia: results of a controlled family study. Arch Gen Psychiatry 50:871–883, 1993

Mednick SA, McNeil T: Current methodology in research on the etiology of schizophrenia. Psychol Bull 70:681–693, 1968

Mills JL, McPartlin JM, Kirke PN, et al: Homocysteine metabolism in pregnancies complicated by neural-tube defects. Lancet 345:149–151, 1995

Mowry BJ, Mamcarrow DJ, Lennon DP, et al: Schizophrenia susceptibility and chromosome 6p24–22. Nat Genet 11:233–234, 1995

O'Callaghan E, Gibson T, Colohan HA, et al: Season of birth in schizophrenia: evidence for confinement of an excess of winter births to patients without a family history of mental disorder. Br J Psychiatry 158:764–769, 1991

Odegaard O: The multifactorial theory of inheritance in predisposition to schizophrenia, in Genetic Factors in Schizophrenia. Edited by Kaplan AR. Springfield, IL, Charles C Thomas, 1972, pp 256–275

Ottman R: Gene–environment interaction: definitions and study designs. Prev Med 25:764–770, 1996

Owens MJ, Lewis SW: Risk factors in schizophrenia (letter). Br J Psychiatry 153:407, 1988

Parnas J, Schulsinger F, Teasdale TW, et al: Perinatal complications and clinical outcome within the schizophrenic spectrum. Br J Psychiatry 140:416–420, 1982

Plomin R: Nature and Nurture: An Introduction to Behavioral Genetics. Pacific Grove, CA, Brooks/Cole, 1990

Prescott CA, Gottesman II: Genetically mediated vulnerability to schizophrenia. Psychiatr Clin North Am 16:245–267, 1993

Pulver AE, Liang KY, Brown CH, et al: Risk factors in schizophrenia: season of birth, gender, and familial risk. Br J Psychiatry 160:65–71, 1992

Pulver AE, Karayiorgou M, Wolyniec PS, et al: Sequential strategy to identify a susceptibility gene for schizophrenia: report of potential linkage on chromosome 22q12–q13.1, part 1. Am J Med Genet 54:36–43, 1995

Rosenthal D: Genetic Theory and Abnormal Behavior. New York, McGraw-Hill, 1970

Rosenthal D, Wender PH, Kety SS, et al: Schizophrenics' offspring reared in adoptive homes. J Psychiatr Res 6:377–391, 1968

Rothman KJ, Greenland S: Modern Epidemiology. Philadelphia, PA, Lippincott-Raven Publishers, 1998

Rudin E: Zur Vererbung und Neuenstehung der Dementia Praecox. Berlin, Springer Verlag, 1916

Schizophrenia Collaborative Group for Chromosomes 3, 6, and 8: A combined analysis of D22S278 marker alleles in affected sib-pairs: support for a susceptibility locus at chromosome 22q12. Am J Med Genet 67: 40–45, 1996

Schwartz S: The role of values in the nature/nurture debate about psychiatric disorders. Social Psychiatry and Psychiatric Epidemiology 8: 356–362, 1998

Shur E: Season of birth in high- and low-risk schizophrenics. Br J Psychiatry 140:410–415, 1982

Solimena M, De Camilli P: Coxsackieviruses and diabetes. Nat Med 1:25–26, 1995

Stabenau JR, Pollin W: Heredity and environment in schizophrenia, revisited: the contribution of twin and high-risk studies. J Nerv Ment Dis 181:290–297, 1993

Stober G, Franzek E, Beckmann H: Pregnancy and labor complications—their significance in the development of schizophrenic psychoses. Fortschr Neurol Psychiatr 61:329–337, 1993

Straub RE, MacLean CJ, O'Neill FA, et al: A potential vulnerability locus for schizophrenia on chromosome 6p24–22: evidence for genetic heterogeneity. Nat Genet 11:287–293, 1995

Straub RE, MacLean CJ, Martin RB, et al: A schizophrenia locus may be located in region 10p15–p11. Am J Med Genet 81:296–301, 1998

Suddath RL, Christison GW, Torrey EF, et al: Anatomical abnormalities in the brains of monozygotic twins discordant for schizophrenia. N Engl J Med 322:789–794, 1990

Sugarman PA, Craufurd D: Schizophrenia in the Afro-Caribbean community. Br J Psychiatry 164:474–480, 1994

Susser ES, Susser M: Genetic epidemiology of psychiatric disorders: examples from schizophrenia, in Psychiatry. Edited by Michaels R. Philadelphia, PA, JB Lippincott, 1992, pp 1–12

Susser E, Brown A, Matte T: Prenatal antecedents of neuropsychiatric disorder over the life course: collaborative studies of US birth cohorts, in Childhood Onset of "Adult" Psychopathology: Clinical and Research Advances. Edited by Rappoport J. Washington, DC, American Psychiatric Press (in press)

Tienari PJ, Wynne LC: Adoption studies of schizophrenia. Ann Med 26:233–237, 1994

Tienari P, Lahti I, Naarald M: Biological mothers in the Finnish adoption study: alternative definitions of schizophrenia. Paper presented at the VIIth World Congress of Psychiatry, Vienna, Austria, July 14, 1983

Tienari P, Wynne LC, Moring J, et al: The Finnish adoptive family study of schizophrenia: implications for family research. Br J Psychiatry (suppl 23):20–26, 1994

Torgersen S, Onstad S, Skre I, et al: "True" schizotypal personality disorder: a study of co-twins and relatives of schizophrenic probands. Am J Psychiatry 150:1661–1667, 1993

van der Put NMJ, Steegers-Theunissen RPM, Frosst P, et al: Mutated methylenetetrahydrofolate reductase as a risk factor for spina bifida. Lancet 346:1070–1071, 1995

Walker E, Hoppes E, Emory E, et al: Environmental factors related to schizophrenia in psychophysiologically liable high-risk males. J Abnorm Psychol 90:313–320, 1981

Wender PH, Rosenthal D, Kety SS, et al: Cross-fostering: a research strategy for clarifying the role of genetic and experiential factors in the etiology of schizophrenia. Arch Gen Psychiatry 30:121–128, 1974

Chapter 3

Prenatal Development of the Brain

Richard S. Nowakowski, Ph.D.

As reviewed by Waddington and colleagues in Chapter 1, evidence is mounting that disruptions of neurodevelopment in the prenatal period could play an etiological role in schizophrenia. Before embarking on an exploration of specific prenatal causes of schizophrenia, it is essential to have a basic understanding of the context in which these early exposures influence brain development. Therefore, the goal of this chapter is to review the early steps of normal development of the brain and the subsequent growth of brain regions that have been implicated in schizophrenia. Readers specifically interested in the epidemiological findings on prenatal risk factors in schizophrenia may proceed, and use this chapter primarily as a reference.

The central nervous system (CNS) abnormalities that accompany schizophrenia include altered morphology and function of the hippocampus and specific cortical regions in the absence of gliosis. Such alterations, which have been demonstrated in both cytoarchitectonic studies (Akbarian et al. 1993; Jakob and Beckmann 1986; Kovelman and Scheibel 1984, 1986) and imaging studies (Bogerts et al. 1993; Shenton et al. 1992; Suddath et al. 1990), are of particular significance, because these brain regions are proposed to be involved in the generation of schizophrenic symptomatology (Besson et al. 1987; Bogerts et al. 1993; Shenton et al. 1992). These findings of altered morphology in areas implicated in schizophrenic symptomatology support the hypothesis that developmental alterations during the prenatal period that involve disruptions in cell proliferation and/or neuronal migration may be an important etiological contributor to schizophrenia and other psychiatric disorders. The goal of this chapter is to review the early steps of normal development of the brain and the subsequent growth of the brain. Special emphasis is given to the general processes of cell proliferation and neuronal migration because of their probable contribution to the etiology of the types of morphological disruptions that accompany schizophrenia and other diseases.

Neurulation and Early Development

The development of the CNS is a complicated, multistep process. Early during the development of a vertebrate embryo, the CNS is formed from the primitive ectoderm in a process known as neurulation (Figure 3–1), the result of which is the neural tube (Figure 3–2). The lumen of the neural tube eventually becomes the ventricular system of the mature brain. The CNS is derived from the neural tube, and the wall of the tube produces and becomes the cells and tissue of the mature brain. The cells just lateral to the edge of the neural plate and some of the cells from the dorsal portion of the neural tube become the neural crest. The neural crest cells produce a variety of structures in the periphery, including most of the peripheral nervous system (LeDouarin 1982).

The neural tube, like any cylindrically shaped object, has three dimensions—longitudinal, circumferential, and radial (see Figure 3–2). Even at the earliest stages, the different portions of the wall of the neural tube have different potentials and, as a result, different fates. As development proceeds, differential differentiation along each of these three dimensions leads to differential expansion of the various subdivisions that is, to a substantial degree, responsible for the diverse anatomy of the mature brain.

The basic organizational plan of the nervous system is defined early during development, predominantly by differentiation along two of the three dimensions, i.e., the length and circumference of the neural tube. Differential differentiation along the longitudinal dimension produces the major subdivisions of the CNS (Figure 3–3). Within the major longitudinal subdivisions are additional seg-

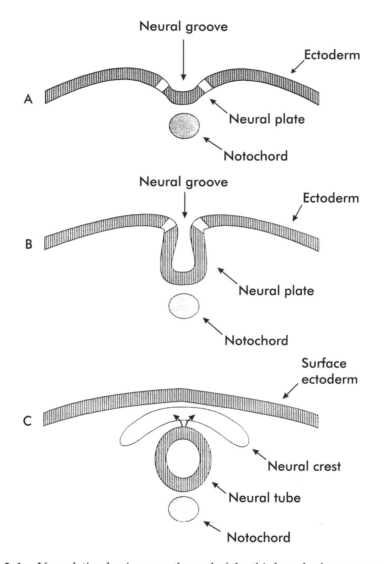

Figure 3–1. Neurulation begins near the end of the third week after conception. The ectoderm, which is the outer surface of the embryo, is induced to fold in upon itself to form the neural tube. *(A)* At the beginning of neurulation, there is a shallow groove just above the notochord; this shallow groove marks the position of the neural plate. *(B)* As the neural groove deepens, the lateral edges of the neural plate fuse *(C)* to become the neural tube. The cells just lateral to the edge of the neural plate and some of the cells from the dorsal portion of the neural tube become the neural crest. The central nervous system is derived from the neural tube. The neural crest cells produce a variety of structures in the periphery, including most of the peripheral nervous system.

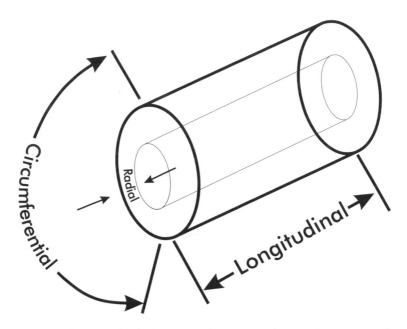

Figure 3–2.   The neural tube has three dimensions: longitudinal, circumferential, and radial. Differentiation along each of these three dimensions proceeds in a different way (see text).

mental subdivisions known as rhombomeres (Lumsden et al. 1994; Nieto et al. 1992). In addition, within each of these major subdivisions, differential differentiation around the neural tube (i.e., in the circumferential dimension) gives rise to the development of structurally and functionally distinct areas.

In the portion of the neural tube that produces the spinal cord, there are four circumferentially defined zones or plates: the roof plate, paired lateral plates, and the floor plate (Figure 3–4A, C). The lateral plate is usually divided by the sulcus limitans into a dorsally positioned alar plate and a ventrally positioned basal plate (Figure 3–4A). The adult spinal cord is derived, for the most part, from the alar and basal plates, which become the dorsal and ventral horns of the spinal cord, respectively (Figure 3–4B).

In more rostral portions of the nervous system (i.e., in the portions of the neural tube that produce the brain stem), the same four circumferential subdivisions exist (i.e., roof, floor, alar, and basal plates); however, differential expansion of the circumferential sub-

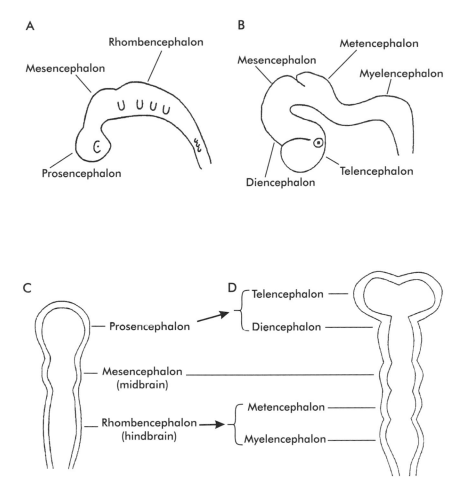

Figure 3–3. Longitudinal differentiation of the neural tube. Differential differentiation along the longitudinal axis produces the major subdivisions of the central nervous system. In a 4-week old human embryo, there are three primary brain vesicles: the prosencephalon, the mesencephalon, and the rhombencephalon *(A, C)*. In the next 2 weeks, the primary vesicles become subdivided. The prosencephalon becomes the telencephalon and the diencephalon, and the rhombencephalon becomes the metencephalon and the myelencephalon *(B, D)*.

divisions produces a significantly different adult morphology in each subdivision of the CNS (Figure 3–4B, D). Specifically, in the medulla the roof plate becomes wide, displacing the alar and basal plates laterally (Figure 3–4C). Thus, in the adult, sensory and motor system derivatives of the alar and basal plates are also pushed aside as a consequence of the expansion of the roof plate and are oriented mediolaterally around the sulcus limitans rather than dorsoventrally as in the spinal cord (Figure 3–4D).

The general significance of this circumferential differentiation is that it precedes the functional organization of the nervous system

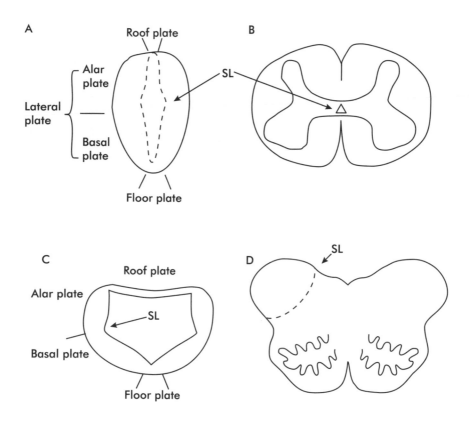

Figure 3–4. Circumferential differentiation of the neural tube. In the spinal cord, there are four circumferential zones, or *plates:* a floor plate, an alar plate, a basal plate, and a roof plate. The names of these plates are derived from their position around the tube (the Latin word *ala* means "wing"). In the medulla, the alar and basal plates are displaced laterally by the widening and attenuation of the roof plate. In both the spinal cord and the medulla, the sulcus limitans (SL) marks the border between the basal and alar plates. In the adult, the morphological relationship between the sensory and motor derivatives of the alar and basal plates is similar, although their orientation around the sulcus limitans shifts from dorsoventral in the spinal cord to mediolateral in the medulla.

into sensory and motor subdivisions. In other parts of the nervous system, such anatomic differentiation also precedes functional differentiation; however, the details of the circumferential compartments differ. A particularly clear example of such anatomic differentiation is in the developing hippocampal region, in which future cytoarchitectonic subdivisions can be detected even as the first neurons that form them are being generated (Nowakowski and Rakic 1979).

The molecular events underlying important portions of these early and basic organizational steps have begun to be elucidated (see reviews by Krumlauf 1994; Placzek 1995; Wilkinson 1993). Future progress in identifying the molecules involved at each step and in each area is certain to lead to advances in the development of diagnostic tests and of methods for therapeutic intervention for numerous neurological and psychiatric disorders.

Cell Proliferation and Neuronal Migration and Differentiation

Additional structural refinement and differentiation in the internal organization of each CNS subdivision is, for the most part, the result of a series of changes in the third dimension of the neural tube, i.e., the radial dimension. The changes in the radial dimension chiefly involve cell proliferation and neuronal migration and differentiation that produce a variety of laminar schemes in different parts of the neural tube. Thus, in order to understand the variety of laminar organizational schemes that exist in the different parts of the adult CNS, it is necessary to understand three distinctly different cellular processes: cell proliferation, neuronal migration, and neuronal differentiation. Although these three processes occur simultaneously within every division and subdivision of the developing CNS, for a single cell these steps represent a cascade of developmental events. In other words, taken together these three steps can be considered to represent the "life history" of a single neuron or glial cell; each cell must pass successively through all three of these steps to become a mature component of the CNS.

Through intercellular interactions, cells present in the same part of the nervous system, in the same or even in different states of maturation, can interact and affect each other's fate. This means that cells that pass through the cascade early can influence the fates of cells subsequently passing through the cascade.

Cell Proliferation

It appears that all of the neurons of the primate CNS are produced during the developmental period, which probably extends only about 3–6 months after birth; there have, however, been reports of neuron production in the adult canary (Goldman and Nottebohm 1983; Nottebohm 1985) and also in the adult rat (Bayer 1982; Bayer et al. 1982; Kaplan 1977; Kaplan and Hinds 1977). For the most part, there is no proliferation of neurons in the adult primate CNS (Nowakowski and Rakic 1981; Rakic 1982, 1985, 1988).

In the developing CNS, cell proliferation occurs within two specialized zones that line the ventricular system (Figure 3–5). The first of these two zones to appear is the ventricular zone (Boulder Committee 1970), which consists of a pseudostratified, columnar epithelium. All parts of the developing CNS have a ventricular zone, and in some parts the ventricular zone is the *only* proliferative zone to appear. In other parts of the developing CNS, a second proliferative zone appears. This zone, known as the subventricular zone, differs in a number of ways from the ventricular zone. The most important of these differences is in the "behavior" of the proliferating cells (Figure 3–5). In the ventricular zone, after each mitotic division the nuclei of the proliferating cells move "to and fro" from the ventricular surface to the border of the ventricular zone with the subventricular zone and back again. The position of the nuclei and the direction of movement are related to the phase of the cell cycle, with mitosis occurring at the ventricular surface and DNA synthesis occurring in the outer half of the ventricular zone (Takahashi et al. 1995a). During development of the mouse neocortex, approximately 11 cell cycles occur over a 6-day period; hence, this to-and-fro movement of the nuclei occurs 11 times (Caviness et al. 1995). With each pass through the cell cycle, an increasing proportion of the daughter cells exit the cell cycle and migrate to the cortex (see below). This proportion increases with each pass through the cell cycle. It has been estimated that the production of the human cortex requires about 33–35 cell cycles instead of the 11 that occur in the mouse (Caviness et al. 1995).

In contrast to the ventricular zone cells, the proliferating subventricular zone cells do not move during the cell cycle, and it is likely that most of the output of the subventricular zone is glial rather than neuronal (Takahashi et al. 1995b). It has been speculated (Nowakowski 1987; Nowakowski and Rakic 1981) that the subventricular zone is a phylogenetically "newer" feature. For example, all of the neurons of the major subdivisions (areas CA1, CA2, and CA3) of the hippocampus, which is classified as an archicortical, or "old," cortical structure, are derived from the ventricular zone (Nowakowski and Rakic 1981). In contrast, a substantial subventricular zone is present in the developing neocortex, and this zone is believed to contribute large numbers of cells to the phylogenetically newer neocortex (Nowakowski and Rakic 1981). A similar developmental scheme appears to exist in the developing diencephalon (Rakic 1977). The early appearance of differences in the distribution of the two proliferative zones along the ventricular surface (Nowakowski and Rakic 1981) indicates that the ventricular surface of the developing nervous system is a mosaic, and that the development of major subdivisions of the CNS follows distinctly different patterns even at early stages. Rakic (1988) has termed this early pattern a *protomap*.

Neuronal Migration

Whereas cell proliferation occurs in areas adjacent to the ventricular surface, neurons in many portions of the adult nervous system are located at quite a distance from the ventricular surface. Therefore, a mechanism for the movement of cells from their site of proliferation to their ultimate position is necessary. There are two basic but very different ways that neurons make this movement. The first is passive cell displacement (Figure 3–6). This type of cell movement does not require active locomotory movement by the

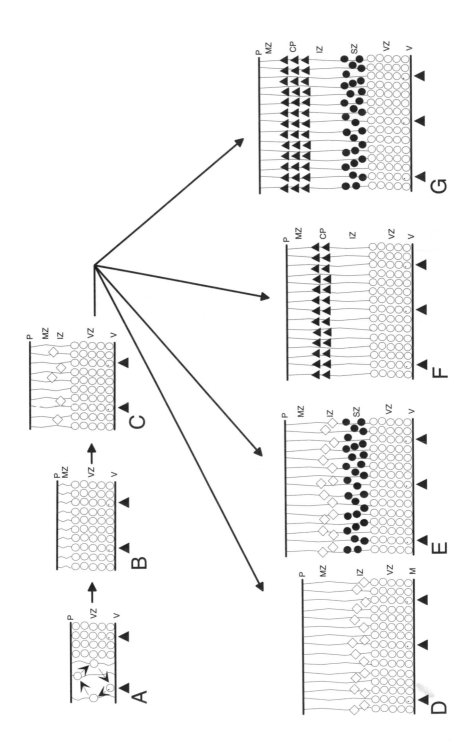

postmitotic neuron. In this case, a postmitotic neuron leaves the proliferative population (influenced to do so by some unknown signal or signals) and is displaced only a very short distance from the border of the proliferative zone. Shortly thereafter, as the next postmitotic neurons are similarly displaced outward from the proliferative zone, the original cells are displaced slightly further.

In those parts of the CNS in which passive cell displacement occurs, neurons that leave the proliferative population the earliest are, in general, those that ultimately are located furthest from the proliferative zone. The subsequently generated neurons are found at levels progressively closer to the proliferative zone (Figure 3–6). Thus, there is a correlation between the final position of a neuron and its time of origin. For areas in which there is passive cell displacement, this correlation is referred to as an "outside to inside"

Figure 3–5.   Radial differentiation in the neural tube. *(A)*, *(B)*, and *(C)* illustrate the early stages of neural tube differentiation. All parts of the early developing central nervous system have a ventricular zone (VZ) and eventually develop a marginal zone (MZ) just subjacent to the pial surface (P). In the VZ, the nuclei of the cells are stratified, but each cell has contacts that reach the ventricular surface (V) and P of the neural tube. The left side of *(A)* illustrates the movement of a single cell as it passes through the various phases of the cell cycle; DNA synthesis occurs in the outer half of the VZ and mitosis (i.e., cell division) occurs adjacent to the V. This movement of the cell's nucleus is known as *interkinetic nuclear migration*. Shortly after neurulation, the neural tube consists only of the VZ. The next zone to appear *(B)* is the MZ, which is an almost cell-free zone just subjacent to the P. Shortly after the formation of the MZ, an intermediate zone (IZ) forms; this zone contains the first postmitotic cells of the nervous system. The IZ is located between the VZ and the MZ. *(D)*, *(E)*, *(F)*, and *(G)* illustrate various alternatives for subsequent radial development of the central nervous system. *(D):* In some parts of the neural tube, the only proliferative zone present is the VZ. The postmitotic cells derived from the VZ aggregate and mature in the IZ, just adjacent to the VZ. One portion of the nervous system that has this pattern of radial differentiation is the spinal cord. *(E):* In other portions of the nervous system, postmitotic cells also aggregate in the IZ and differentiate there, but some of these cells are derived from the subventricular zone (SZ). The dorsal thalamus is an example of a portion of the nervous system that follows this pattern of development. *(F)* and *(G)* are examples of cortical regions. In the hippocampus *(F)*, all of the postmitotic cells are derived from the VZ. They migrate across the sparsely populated IZ and form a cortical plate (CP). In the neocortex *(G)*, both a VZ and an SZ are present. Again, the derivatives of these two proliferative zones migrate across the IZ and form a CP.

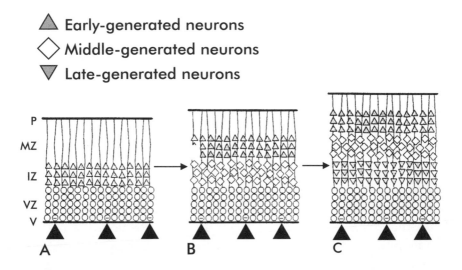

△ Early-generated neurons
◇ Middle-generated neurons
▽ Late-generated neurons

Figure 3–6.   In some areas of the developing nervous system, cell movement occurs via passive displacement. Some cells leave the proliferative zone and take up a position only a short distance away. Later, as other cells are produced by the proliferative zone, the earlier-produced cells are displaced outward. *(A)* through *(C)* illustrate the progressive passive displacement of previously generated neurons away from the ventricular surface (V) by subsequently generated neurons. *(A):* The earliest-generated neurons that leave the ventricular zone (VZ) are represented as *triangles*. *(B):* The next group of neurons to be generated are represented by *diamonds*. Their movement out of the VZ displaces the earlier-generated neurons toward the pial surface (P). *(C):* The last neurons generated *(inverted triangles)* displace both of the earlier-generated populations of neurons. This sequence of events produces a specific distribution of neurons known as an *outside-to-inside* spatiotemporal gradient. IZ = intermediate zone; MZ = marginal zone.

spatiotemporal gradient. Outside and inside are both defined with respect to the position of the cells relative to the proliferative zone; for the most part, *outside* refers to the pial surface, and *inside* refers to the ventricular surface. Areas of the nervous system in which the outside-to-inside spatiotemporal gradient is manifest include the thalamus (Altman and Bayer 1979; Angevine 1970; Rakic 1977), the hypothalamus (Ifft 1972), the spinal cord (Nornes and Das 1974), many regions of the brain stem (Altman and Bayer 1981; Taber-Pierce 1972), the retina (Sidman 1961; Walsh et al. 1983), and the dentate gyrus of the hippocampal formation (Angevine 1965; Bayer

1982; Bayer et al. 1982; Nowakowski and Rakic 1981; Wyss and Sripanidkulchai 1985).

The second way that young neurons move from the proliferative zone to their ultimate positions is neuronal migration (for a review, see Sidman and Rakic 1973). This process takes place in the cerebral cortex (both archicortex and neocortex) and requires the active participation of the postmitotic neurons in producing their own displacement. Migrating neurons leave the proliferative zone and move a great distance through the intermediate zone and cortical plate, and as a result, progressively later-generated neurons bypass earlier-produced ones (Figure 3–7).

In those parts of the developing CNS in which the migrating young neurons actively contribute to their own displacement away from the proliferative zones, the result is an "inside to outside" spatiotemporal gradient. In this pattern, the earliest-generated cells remain closest to the proliferative zone and form the deepest layers, while the latest-generated cells move farthest from the proliferative zone and occupy the most superficial layers. Inside-to-outside spatiotemporal gradients are found in most portions of the cerebral cortex (Angevine 1965; Angevine and Sidman 1961; Caviness 1982; Caviness and Sidman 1973; Hinds 1968; Miller 1985, 1987; Rakic 1975b; Rakic and Nowakowski 1981; Wyss and Sripanidkulchai 1985) and in several subcortical areas (Cooper and Rakic 1981; Hickey and Hitchcock 1968). Areas in which spatiotemporal gradients of the inside-to-outside type occur are, in general, well-laminated structures in that they have tangentially oriented layers that run parallel with the surface of the proliferative zones. During migration, many neurons are guided to their final position by radial glial fibers (Rakic 1971, 1972), which provide the scaffolding for the future adult neocortex and for other cortical and noncortical structures as well (Eckenhoff and Rakic 1984; Nowakowski and Rakic 1979; Rakic 1971, 1978, 1982; Rakic et al. 1974). It has also been speculated that radial glial fibers provide the scaffolding for the columnar organization of the adult cortex (Eckenhoff and Rakic 1984; Mountcastle 1978; Rakic 1978, 1982, 1988; Smart and McSherry 1982).

The process of neuronal migration (Figure 3–8) is a complicated

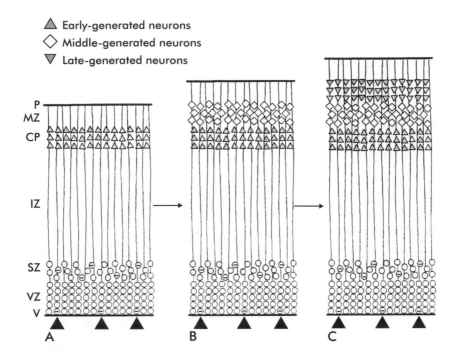

Figure 3–7. The sequence of events associated with active neuronal migration. In some parts of the developing central nervous system, neurons leaving the proliferative zone move a great distance before taking up their final position. *(A):* The first neurons to leave the proliferative zone *(triangles)* assemble in a formation known as a cortical plate (CP), which is situated between the intermediate zone (IZ) and the marginal zone (MZ). *(B):* The next group of neurons to be generated *(diamonds)* leaves the proliferative population and moves across the IZ and past the earlier-generated cells to take up a position on the top of the CP. *(C):* The last-generated neurons *(inverted triangles)* migrate across the intermediate zone and past both groups of earlier-generated cells to take up residence at the top of the CP. This type of distribution of neurons is known as an *inside-to-outside* spatiotemporal gradient. P = pial surface; SZ = subventricular zone; V = ventricular surface; VZ = ventricular zone.

one and consists of at least three phases (for a review, see Nowa-kowski 1985): an initiation phase, a locomotory phase, and a termination phase. In the initiation phase, a young neuron starts its migration by leaving the proliferative population; during this phase, a cell in the proliferating population makes the transition from neuroblast (i.e., a proliferating cell) to young neuron (i.e., a nonproliferating, permanently postmitotic cell). The young neuron

Stages of neuronal migration

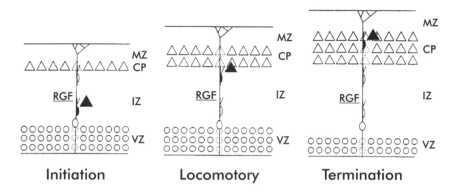

Initiation   Locomotory   Termination

Figure 3–8.   Schematic illustration of the interaction between migrating neurons and radial glial fibers (RGFs). After leaving the proliferative zone, the young neuron is guided by a radially aligned glial cell as it moves toward its final position in the cortical plate (CP). The progression of one such young neuron *(black cell marked by arrow)* from the proliferative zone through the intermediate zone (IZ) to the CP is illustrated. The migratory process can be divided into three stages. In the early stage, the young neuron leaves the proliferative population, becomes apposed to an RGF, and acquires a polarity directed toward the pial surface (P). In the middle stage, the neuron enters the locomotory phase and traverses the IZ, maintaining its apposition to the RGF and its polarity as it moves through the zone. In the late stage, the neuron reaches the top of the CP, loses its apposition to the RGF, and reorganizes its polarity in order to differentiate into a mature neuron. Disruption of any of the three steps of the migratory process can result in *ectopic neurons,* i.e., neurons in the "wrong" position. MZ = marginal zone; VZ = ventricular zone.

becomes apposed to a radial glial fiber and establishes an axis of polarity away from the ventricular surface. Once the neuron is aligned with the radial glial fiber, the second, or locomotory, phase of migration begins. During this phase, the young neuron moves actively along the surface of a radial glial cell, retaining both its apposition to the radial glial fiber and its axis of polarity away from the proliferative zone. In the cerebral cortex, the locomotory phase can be very long: a migrating neuron can move along a radial glial fiber that may be tens of millimeters long. The termination phase of neuronal migration occurs when the migrating young neuron reaches the vicinity of its final position. At this point, the neuron must stop its migration and become detached from the radial glial fiber. It then can continue its differentiation process by growing dendrites and sending out axons that eventually make contacts with other neurons.

Neuronal Differentiation

The final phase in the life history of a neuron is differentiation. This is an extraordinarily complex process that is responsible for a large proportion of the cellular and functional diversity of the neurons of the adult CNS. The process of cell differentiation in the CNS, as outlined briefly below, is quite complex, and a full discussion is beyond the scope of this chapter.

During the differentiation of a neuron, axonal and dendritic processes are elaborated, and neurotransmitter phenotypes are expressed. In many cases, the axon grows a long distance over a complicated terrain until it reaches its final target. The dendrites grow out and form a characteristic arborization pattern for each particular cell class. The specific neurotransmitter enzymes that are characteristic of that cell class are also produced. In addition to elaborating the specific enzymes to produce neurotransmitters, a neuron must also produce at each postsynaptic site the specific receptors it needs to receive input from its various presynaptic partners. Also, some neurons will die, apparently as a result of failing to establish appropriate connections.

As neurons are acquiring their mature properties, glial cells produced in the subventricular zone become more numerous and also differentiate into various forms; some become oligodendrocytes that produce myelin, others become astrocytes that perform other functions (ffrench-Constant and Raff 1986; Temple and Raff 1986). In humans, it is known that myelination of most pathways in the CNS continues long after birth (for a review, see Richardson 1982). In fact, Flechsig (1920), in his classic work on myelination in the developing human cerebral cortex, established the basis of the traditional classification of neocortical areas into primary, secondary, and association cortices.

Clinicopathological Correlates

If any of the three phases involved in neuronal migration are disrupted, an abnormality in cell position results. Neurons that fail to reach their appropriate positions are said to be ectopic (or heterotopic) (Rakic 1975a). Neuropathologists have described a variety of defects in cell position. In humans, the best-studied examples of defects in neuronal positioning are in the cerebral cortex, where abnormalities in neuronal migration have been associated with a variety of diseases and syndromes ranging from extremely severe mental retardation and failure to thrive to behavioral disorders. Two behavioral disorders that have been associated with the disruption of the migratory process are schizophrenia and dyslexia. In the case of schizophrenia, there is evidence for the existence of ectopic neurons in the hippocampus and elsewhere in the temporolimbic cortex in the brains of patients with severe schizophrenia (Akbarian et al. 1993; Jakob and Beckmann 1986; Kovelman and Scheibel 1984, 1986). In the case of dyslexia, Galaburda and colleagues (1983) found islands of ectopic neurons in the brains of several individuals with a severe form of the disorder. In addition, a number of more severe disorders associated with disruptions of the migratory process include hydrocephalus, methanol exposure, mental retardation, seizures, lissencephaly, methylmercury poisoning, exposure to radiation, and craniofacial anomalies (Choi and Kudo 1981; Choi et al. 1978; Evrard et al. 1978; Mikhael and Mattar 1978; Miller 1986; Otake and Schull 1984; Richman et al. 1975; Zimmerman et al. 1983).

From human pathological data, at present it is not possible to determine the developmental fate of neurons that fail to migrate to their proper positions and the functional modifications that may or may not result. Do these abnormally positioned neurons make connections with the rest of the brain, and, if so, do they make connections with their normal targets or with other targets? Perhaps even more importantly, it is not known how these abnormalities in connectivity (if they exist) might affect the function of the areas of the brain in which these cells were originally destined to reside.

Studies in mutant mice may begin to provide some of the answers to these questions. Defects in neuronal migration in these mice clearly show that ectopic neurons do make connections with other normally positioned constituents of the nervous system (Caviness and Rakic 1978; Nowakowski 1988; Sekiguchi et al. 1993, 1994, 1995). Recently, investigators have cloned the *LIS1* gene, which produces Miller-Dieker lissencephaly and probably has a role in neuronal migration (Hattori et al. 1994; Reiner et al. 1995). This advance will enable researchers to produce knockout and transgenic mice,[1] thereby making available molecularly authentic murine analogues of the human disease. The use of such animal models promises to delineate the structural and functional alterations that result from neuronal migration disturbances, findings with potentially important implications for our understanding of the etiopathogenic processes that occur in schizophrenia.

Summary and Conclusions

The normal development of the human CNS follows a programmed, orderly, and progressive cascade of events. Beginning with neurulation, which leads to the formation of the neural tube, the subsequent anatomic and functional organization of the nervous system unfolds via differential differentiation along each of three dimensions: longitudinal, circumferential, and radial. Structural refinement and differentiation is accomplished through three major sequential processes: cell proliferation, neuronal migration, and neuronal differentiation. During the period of cell proliferation, which is believed to end 3–6 months after birth, all of the neurons of the primate CNS are produced. Cell proliferation occurs in two specialized zones lining the ventricular system: a ventricular zone and, in some regions, a subventricular zone. Neurons move from their site of proliferation to their ultimate destination through

---

[1] In a knockout mouse, a specific gene is removed; the resulting phenotype is used to analyze the function of the gene. In a transgenic mouse, an "extra" foreign gene is added to the genome and the gene product is then produced in excess in or in an abnormal position; the resulting phenotype provides a different perspective on the gene's function. Thus, these powerful tools of molecular biology provide a crucial link between genetics and gene functions.

passive cell displacement and neuronal migration, which follow two different and respective spatiotemporal gradients: "outside to inside" and "inside to outside." Neuronal migration involves three phases: an initiation phase, a locomotory phase in which the neuron moves along a radial glial fiber, and a termination phase. During neuronal differentiation, the last period in neuronal development, elaboration of axonal and dendritic processes occurs, neurotransmitter phenotypes are expressed, and axons are myelinated.

An understanding of normal developmental processes provides an important framework on which to conceptualize the mechanisms whereby prenatal exposures may interfere with brain maturation. Disruptions at any point of this developmental cascade may result from a variety of prenatal insults, including ionizing radiation, nutritional deprivation, and prenatal infection. As elaborated later in this volume (see Chapters 4, 5, and 6), the latter two of these insults have been associated with schizophrenia.

Ectopic neurons, which are present in schizophrenia and other neuropsychiatric disorders, are likely the result of disruptions of neuronal migration. In addition, the increased ventricular size, reflecting presumably decreased cerebral volume, is likely the result of either a reduction in neuronal production or an increase in neuronal cell death. All of these events occur during the second trimester. Thus, it is tempting to speculate that the second-trimester specificity of influenza epidemics on schizophrenia is related to specific disruptions of cell proliferation, neuronal migration, and/or neuronal cell death. It is even possible that disruptions of these developmental processes, i.e., different etiologies, could produce similar functional disturbances.

References

Akbarian S, Vineula A, Kim JJ, et al: Distorted distribution of nicotinamide–adenine dinucleotide phosphate–diaphorase neurons in temporal lobe of schizophrenics implies anomalous cortical development. Arch Gen Psychiatry 50:178–187, 1993

Altman J, Bayer SA: Development of the diencephalon in the rat, V: thy-midine-radiographic observations on internuclear and intranuclear gradients in the thalamus. J Comp Neurol 188:473–500, 1979

Altman J, Bayer SA: Development of the brain stem in the rat, V: thy-midine-radiographic study of the time of origin of neurons in the midbrain tegmentum. J Comp Neurol 198:677–716, 1981

Angevine JB Jr: Time of neuron origin in the hippocampal region: an autoradiographic study in the mouse. Exp Neurol 2 (suppl):1–71, 1965

Angevine JB Jr: Time of neuron origin in the diencephalon of the mouse: an autoradiographic study. J Comp Neurol 139:129–188, 1970

Angevine JB Jr, Sidman RL: Autoradiographic study of cell migration during histogenesis of cerebral cortex in the mouse. Nature 192:766–768, 1961

Bayer SA: Changes in the total number of dentate granule cells in juvenile and adult rats: a correlated volumetric and [³H]thymidine autoradio-graphic study. Exp Brain Res 46:315–323, 1982

Bayer SA, Yackel JW, Puri PS: Neurons in the rat dentate gyrus granular layer substantially increase during juvenile and adult life. Science 216: 890–892, 1982

Besson JAO, Corrigan FM, Cherryman GR, et al: Nuclear magnetic resonance brain imaging in chronic schizophrenia. Br J Psychiatry 150: 161–163, 1987

Bogerts B, Lieberman JA, Ashtari M, et al: Hippocampus-amygdala volumes and psychopathology in chronic schizophrenia. Biol Psychiatry 33:236–246, 1993

Boulder Committee: Embryonic vertebrate central nervous system: revised terminology. Anat Rec 166:257–261, 1970

Caviness VS Jr: Neocortical histogenesis in normal and reeler mice: a developmental study based on [³H]thymidine autoradiography. Brain Res 256:293–302, 1982

Caviness VS Jr, Rakic P: Mechanisms of cortical development: a view from mutations in mice. Annu Rev Neurosci 1:297–326, 1978

Caviness VS Jr, Sidman RL: Time of origin of corresponding cell classes in the cerebral cortex of normal and reeler mutant mice: an autoradiographic analysis. J Comp Neurol 148:141–152, 1973

Caviness VS Jr, Takahashi T, Nowakowski RS: Numbers, time and neocortical neuronogenesis: a general developmental and evolutionary model. Trends Neurosci 18:379–383, 1995

Choi BH, Kudo M: Abnormal migration and gliomatosis in epidermal nevus syndrome. Acta Neuropathol 53:319–325, 1981

Choi BH, Lapham LW, Amin-Zaki L, et al: Abnormal neuronal migration, deranged cerebral cortical organization, and diffuse white matter astrocytosis of human fetal brain: a major effect of methylmercury poisoning in utero. J Neuropathol Exp Neurol 37:719–733, 1978

Cooper ML, Rakic P: Neurogenetic gradients in the superior and inferior colliculi of the rhesus monkey. J Comp Neurol 202:309–334, 1981

Eckenhoff MF, Rakic P: Radial organization of the hippocampal dentate gyrus: a Golgi, ultrastructural and immunocytochemical analysis in the developing rhesus monkey. J Comp Neurol 223:1–21, 1984

Evrard P, Caviness VS Jr, Prats-Vinas J, et al: The mechanism of arrest of neuronal migration in the Zellweger malformation: an hypothesis based upon cytoarchitectonic analysis. Acta Neuropathol 41:109–117, 1978

ffrench-Constant C, Raff MC: Proliferating bipotential glial progenitor cells in adult rat optic nerve. Nature 319:499–502, 1986

Flechsig P: Anatomie des menschlichen Gehirns und Ruckenmarks auf myelogenetischer Grundlage. Leipzig, Germany, Georg Theime, 1920

Galaburda AM, Sherman GF, Geschwind N: Developmental dyslexia: third consecutive case with cortical anomalies. Society for Neuroscience Abstracts 9:940, 1983

Goldman SA, Nottebohm F: Neuronal production, migration, and differentiation in a vocal control nucleus of the adult female canary brain. Proc Natl Acad Sci U S A 80:2390–2394, 1983

Hattori MH, Adachi M, Tsujimoto H, et al: Miller-Dieker lissencephaly gene encodes a subunit of brain platelet-activating factor. Nature 370: 216–218, 1994

Hickey TL, Hitchcock PF: Neurogenesis in the cat lateral geniculate nucleus: a [^{3}H]thymidine study. J Comp Neurol 228:186–199, 1968

Hinds JW: Autoradiographic study of histogenesis in the mouse olfactory bulb, I: time of origin of neurons and neuroglia. J Comp Neurol 134: 287–304, 1968

Ifft JD: An autoradiographic study of the time of final division of neurons in the rat hypothalamic nuclei. J Comp Neurol 144:193–204, 1972

Jakob H, Beckmann H: Prenatal developmental disturbances in the limbic allocortex in schizophrenics. J Neural Transm 65:303–326, 1986

Kaplan MS: Neurogenesis in the 3-month-old rat visual cortex. J Comp Neurol 195:323–338, 1977

Kaplan MS, Hinds JW: Neurogenesis in the adult rat: electron microscopic analysis of light radioautographs. Science 197:1092–1094, 1977

Kovelman JA, Scheibel AB: A neurohistological correlate of schizophrenia. Biol Psychiatry 19:1601–1621, 1984

Kovelman JA, Scheibel AB: Biological substrates of schizophrenia. Acta Neurol Scand 73:1–32, 1986

Krumlauf R: *Hox* genes in vertebrate development. Cell 78:191–201, 1994

LeDouarin N: The Neural Crest. Cambridge, England, Cambridge University Press, 1982

Lumsden JD, Clarke R, Keynes S, et al: Early phenotypic choices by neuronal precursors, revealed by clonal analysis of the chick embryo hindbrain. Development 1208:1581–1589, 1994

Mikhael MA, Mattar AG: Malformation of the cerebral cortex with heterotopia of the gray matter. J Comput Assist Tomogr 2:291–296, 1978

Miller MW: Cogeneration of retrogradely labeled corticocortical projection and GABA-immunoreactive local circuit neurons in cerebral cortex. Developmental Brain Research 23:187–192, 1985

Miller MW: Effects of alcohol on the generation and migration of cerebral cortical neurons. Science 233:1308–1311, 1986

Miller MW: The effect of prenatal exposure to alcohol on the distribution and the time of origin of corticospinal neurons in the rat. J Comp Neurol 257:372–382, 1987

Mountcastle VB: An organizing principle for cerebral function: the unit module and distributed system, in The Mindful Brain. Edited by Edelman G, Mountcastle VB. Cambridge, MA, MIT Press, 1978, pp 7–50

Nieto MA, Bradley LC, Hunt P, et al: Molecular mechanisms of pattern formation in the vertebrate hindbrain. Ciba Found Symp 165:92–102, 1992

Nornes HL, Das GD: Temporal patterns of neurons in spinal cord of rat, I: an autoradiographic study—time and sites of origin and migration and settling pattern of neuroblasts. Brain Res 73:121–138, 1974

Nottebohm F: Neuronal replacement in adulthood. Ann N Y Acad Sci 457:143–161, 1985

Nowakowski RS: Neuronal migration in the hippocampal lamination defect (Hld) mutant mouse, in Cellular and Molecular Control of Direct Cell Interactions. Edited by Marthy HJ. New York, Plenum, 1985, pp 133–154

Nowakowski RS: Basic concepts of CNS development. Child Dev 58:568–595, 1987

Nowakowski RS: Development of the hippocampal formation in mutant mice. Drug Development Research 15:315–336, 1988

Nowakowski RS, Rakic P: The mode of migration of neurons to the hippocampus: a Golgi and electron microscopic analysis in foetal rhesus monkey. J Neurocytol 8:697–718, 1979

Nowakowski RS, Rakic P: The site of origin and route and rate of migration of neurons to the hippocampal region of the rhesus monkey. J Comp Neurol 196:129–154, 1981

Otake M, Schull WJ: In utero exposure to A-bomb radiation and mental retardation: a reassessment. Br J Radiol 57:409–414, 1984

Placzek M: The role of the notochord and floor plate in inductive interactions. Curr Opin Genet Dev 5:499–506, 1995

Rakic P: Neuron-glia relationship during granule cell migration in developing cerebellar cortex: a Golgi and electron microscopic study in *Macacus rhesus.* J Comp Neurol 141:283–312, 1971

Rakic P: Mode of migration to the superficial layers of fetal monkey neocortex. J Comp Neurol 145:61–83, 1972

Rakic P: Cell migration and neuronal ectopias in the brain. Birth Defects: Original Article Series 11:95–129, 1975a

Rakic P: Timing of major ontogenetic events in the visual cortex of the rhesus monkey, in Brain Mechanisms in Mental Retardation. New York, Academic Press, 1975b, pp 3–40

Rakic P: Genesis of the dorsal lateral geniculate nucleus in the rhesus monkey: site and time of origin, kinetics of proliferation, routes of migration and pattern of distribution of neurons. J Comp Neurol 176:23–52, 1977

Rakic P: Neuronal migration and contact guidance in the primate telencephalon. Postgrad Med J 54 (suppl 1):25–40, 1978

Rakic P: Early developmental events: cell lineages, acquisition of neuronal positions, and areal and laminar development. Neurosciences Research Program Bulletin 20:439–451, 1982

Rakic P: Limits of neurogenesis in primates. Science 227:1054–1056, 1985

Rakic P: Specification of cerebral cortical areas. Science 241:170–176, 1988

Rakic P, Nowakowski RS: The time of origin of neurons in the hippocampal region of the rhesus monkey. J Comp Neurol 196:99–128, 1981

Rakic P, Stensaas LJ, Sayre EP, et al: Computer-aided three-dimensional reconstruction and quantitative analysis of cells from serial electron microscopic montages of foetal monkey brain. Nature 250:31–34, 1974

Reiner O, Albrecht U, Gordon M, et al: Lissencephaly gene (*LIS1*) expression in the CNS suggests a role in neuronal migration. J Neurosci 15: 3730–3738, 1995

Richardson EP Jr: Myelination in the human central nervous system, in Histology and Histopathology of the Nervous System, Vol 1. Edited by Haymaker W, Adams RD. Springfield, IL, Charles C Thomas, 1982, pp 146–173

Richman DP, Stewart RM, Hutchinson JW, et al: Mechanical model of brain convolutional development. Science 189:18–21, 1975

Sekiguchi M, Nowakowski RS, Shimai K, et al: Abnormal distribution of acetylcholinesterase activity in the hippocampal formation of the dreher mutant mouse. Brain Res 622:203–210, 1993

Sekiguchi M, Abe H, Shimai K, et al: Disruption of neuronal migration in the neocortex of the dreher mutant mouse. Developmental Brain Research 77:37–43, 1994

Sekiguchi M, Nowakowski RS, Nagato Y, et al: Morphological abnormalities in the hippocampus of the weaver mutant mouse. Brain Res 696: 262–267, 1995

Shenton ME, Kikinis R, Jolescz FA, et al: Abnormalities of the left temporal lobe and thought disorder in schizophrenia: a quantitative magnetic resonance imaging study. N Engl J Med 327:604–612, 1992

Sidman RL: Histogenesis of mouse retina studied with thymidine-H3, in Structure of the Eye. Edited by Smelser G. New York, Academic Press, 1961, pp 487–506

Sidman RL, Rakic P: Neuronal migration with special reference to developing human brain: a review. Brain Res 62:1–35, 1973

Smart IHM, McSherry GM: Growth patterns in the lateral wall of the mouse telencephalon, II: histological changes during and subsequent to the period of isocortical neuron production. J Anat 134:415–442, 1982

Suddath RL, Christison GW, Torrey EF, et al: Anatomical abnormalities in the brains of monozygotic twins discordant for schizophrenia. N Engl J Med 322:789–794, 1990

Taber-Pierce E: Time of origin of neurons in the brain stem of the mouse. Prog Brain Res 40:53–66, 1972

Takahashi T, Nowakowski RS, Caviness VS Jr: The cell cycle of the pseudostratified epithelium of the embryonic murine cerebral wall. J Neurosci 15:6046–6057, 1995a

Takahashi T, Nowakowski RS, Caviness VS Jr: Early ontogeny of the secondary population of the embryonic murine cerebral wall. J Neurosci 15:6058–6068, 1995b

Temple S, Raff MC: Clonal analysis of oligodendrocyte development in culture: evidence for a developmental clock that counts cell divisions. Cell 44:773–779, 1986

Walsh C, Polley EH, Hickey TL, et al: Generation of cat retinal ganglion cells in relation to central pathways. Nature 302:611–614, 1983

Wilkinson DG: Molecular mechanisms of segmental patterning in the vertebrate hindbrain. Perspect Dev Neurobiol 1:117–125, 1993

Wyss JM, Sripanidkulchai B: The development of Ammon's horn and the fascia dentata in the cat: a [³H]thymidine analysis. Developmental Brain Research 18:185–198, 1985

Zimmerman RA, Bilaniuk LT, Grossman RI: Computed tomography in migratory disorders of human brain development. Neuroradiology 25:257–263, 1983

Part II

Prenatal Infectious Exposures

Chapter 4

Seasonality, Prenatal Influenza Exposure, and Schizophrenia

Padraig Wright, M.R.C.Psych., Noriyoshi Takei, M.D., M.Sc.,
Robin M. Murray, D.Sc., F.R.C.Psych., and
Pak C. Sham, M.R.C.Psych.

The single most powerful known risk factor for schizophrenia is being related to a person with schizophrenia (Gottesman 1991). The results of several studies indicate that this risk is increased if the affected relative is female (Bellodi et al. 1986; Goldstein 1992; Wolyniec et al. 1992) or has developed schizophrenia during adolescence or early adulthood (Gordon et al. 1994; Sham et al. 1994). The inherited, and presumably genetic, contribution to the etiology of schizophrenia thus appears to be greatest for female probands with early-onset disease.

Heredity is said to explain 70% of the liability to schizophrenia in some populations (Kendler 1983; McGuffin et al. 1994; Rao et al. 1981), but the precise mode of inheritance is obscure and clearly non-Mendelian. Gottesman and Shields (1982) has suggested that schizophrenia is probably caused by multiple genetic and environmental factors of varying effect size and frequency. Similarly, Kendler (1983) has stated that although nongenetic factors may account for only a small proportion of the variance in liability to schizophrenia in many populations, such factors are nonetheless certainly involved. Current etiological research therefore aims to identify genes and/or environmental factors that are either common or of large effect, or both.

The genetics of schizophrenia have been reviewed many times

(e.g., McGuffin et al. 1995), and several candidate environmental agents have been proposed and investigated, ranging from birth injury (S. W. Lewis and Murray 1987) to cannabis abuse (McGuire et al. 1994) (see other chapters in this volume). In this chapter we discuss prenatal influenza exposure, a postulated environmental factor that is the focus of much contemporary research and controversy.

Is There a "Schizovirus"?

The idea of a possible association between schizophrenia and infectious disease is not new. Kraepelin (1919), no doubt encouraged by the endemic nature of many infections during the early decades of this century, considered that "infections in the years of development might have a causal significance" for schizophrenia, and a range of causative infections were proposed, including tuberculosis (Gosline 1919), typhus, cholera and influenza (Skliar 1922), and syphilis (Gosline 1917). In 1928, Menninger described 67 cases of dementia praecox in a group of 175 patients whose mental illness he believed to have been caused by influenza contracted during the 1919 pandemic. He almost predicted the current debate about the nature of the relationship between influenza and schizophrenia when he wrote that "the psychotic picture revealed in a particular case by a toxic attack on the encephalon probably depends on the kind of mental substructure preexisting, and not demonstrably on the kind of toxin or infection" (Menninger 1928, p. 479), and further stated that "influenza is the only acute febrile disease which occurs with sufficient ubiquity and morbidity to make possible any general statistical study of its psychic effects" (Menninger 1928, p. 468). However, more than 40 years were to pass before infectious agents again assumed interest for schizophrenia researchers. This resurgence of interest occurred because of the discovery of slow virus diseases, and the observation that an excess of schizophrenic patients had been born during late winter and spring (Hare et al. 1972; Machon et al. 1983).

In 1972 the slow virus diseases of kuru and Creutzfeldt-Jakob dementia were described (Gibbs and Gajdusek 1972). The following year, Torrey (1973) suggested that schizophrenia might be due to a slow virus (later whimsically termed the "schizovirus" by his colleagues [Torrey 1988]) and proposed that serum, cerebrospinal fluid (CSF), and brain tissue from schizophrenic patients should be examined for viral antigens and antibodies. This work has been undertaken both by Torrey's own group and by other researchers, who have studied candidate pathogens such as cytomegalovirus (Torrey et al. 1982), herpes virus (Libikova et al. 1979), and retroviruses (Crow 1984) and have produced a conflicting array of results (for a review, see Wright and Murray 1993 and Wright et al. 1993). Most recently, Sierra-Honigmann and colleagues (1995), using polymerase chain reaction analysis, were unable to detect nucleic acids coding for cytomegalovirus, human immunodeficiency virus, influenza A virus, Borna disease virus, or bovine viral diarrhea pestivirus in hippocampal tissue, CSF, and mononuclear leukocytes from schizophrenic patients. These authors concluded that "in these patients schizophrenia is not associated with a persistent or latent infection due to these viruses" (Sierra-Honigmann et al. 1995, p. 59). However, in a study of monozygotic twin pairs discordant for schizophrenia, Yolken et al. (1993) reported a significantly higher frequency of pestivirus antibody in the affected individuals compared with their unaffected co-twins.

Can the Season-of-Birth Effect be Explained?

The season-of-birth effect in schizophrenia remains to be explained. Of the more than 50 studies that have examined the birthdates of schizophrenic patients in the Northern Hemisphere, the majority report that a 5%–15% excess of patients are born between January and March (Boyd et al. 1986; Bradbury and Miller 1985; Pallast et al. 1994); much less remarked upon but perhaps of equal importance is the deficit of schizophrenic births in the late summer and autumn. Southern Hemisphere research has been less extensive, and some studies there have not detected a season-of-birth effect (e.g., Jones and Frei 1979). However, Dalen (1975) in South Africa and Parker and Neilson (1976) in Australia have reported an excess of schizophrenic females born between May and October. In Queensland, Australia, immigrant schizophrenic patients who were born in the Northern Hemisphere show an excess of births in the first two quarters of the year, while an excess of similar magnitude for Australian-born schizophrenic patients occurs in the second and third quarters of the year (Welham et al. 1993).

Two methodological artifacts have been proposed to explain these apparently well-replicated findings. The *age incidence effect* is based on the fact that new cases of schizophrenia increase in incidence during the second 15 years of an individual's life (Hare et al. 1974). If age is determined in whole years on the basis of the calendar year of birth, it follows that individuals born during the first few months of any year will be older in real terms than those born later in the year; they will therefore have experienced a longer period at risk of developing schizophrenia. The *age prevalence effect* stems from the fact that the risk of schizophrenia increases cumulatively with age (S. W. Lewis 1989; M. S. Lewis and Griffin 1981). Individuals born during the early months of a year not only will have had longer absolute risk exposure but also, being older, will have spent more time in a higher-risk period of life, and will therefore have higher rates of illness than those born later in the year. However, contemporary researchers who have applied statistical corrections for the age incidence and age prevalence effects (Pallast et al. 1994) or who have calculated age by month of birth (O'Callaghan et al. 1991a) continue to report a season-of-birth effect on the order of 10%–15%. Southern Hemisphere studies are not subject to either the age incidence or the age prevalence effect because the seasons of interest do not occur in the early part of the year, and research such as that reported by Welham and colleagues (1993) is thus of particular value.

If the season-of-birth effect is not a statistical artifact, how may it be explained? Although several explanations have been put forward, there are two principal hypotheses: 1) mothers of schizophrenic patients have an unusual pattern of conception, and 2) birth during the colder months of the year allows exposure of the unborn fetus or neonate to an unknown environmental factor that increases risk for schizophrenia.

We are aware of six major studies that have examined the hypothesis that mothers of schizophrenic patients have an unusual pattern of conception; four of these studies reported negative results (Buck and Simpson 1978; Machon et al. 1983; Pulver et al. 1992; Watson et al. 1984) and two reported positive results (Hare 1976; McNeil et al. 1976). Of these six reports, perhaps the study by Pulver's group had the best design. They tested the hypothesis that birthdates of the siblings of winter-born schizophrenic patients (401 siblings of 120 winter/spring-born schizophrenic patients) would show an unusual distribution, similar to that of the probands themselves; however, they found that such siblings were no more likely to be born in the winter or spring than the siblings of healthy winter/spring-born control subjects.

It thus appears probable that the season-of-birth effect in schizophrenia is attributable neither to a methodological artifact nor to unusual patterns of conception in the mothers of schizophrenic patients. This suggests the need to search for a seasonally varying environmental factor that adversely affects either fetuses in utero destined to be born in late winter and spring or neonates actually born during these two seasons.

Is There Evidence That Influenza and Schizophrenia Are Associated?

In 1980, Wrede and colleagues, in the course of a prospective study of the offspring of schizophrenic mothers in Finland, concluded that viral infection during fetal development might be an important cause of the perinatal disturbances that were associated with both enlarged cerebral ventricles and schizophrenia (Wrede et al. 1980). Based on the season-of-birth literature, this group subsequently carried out a study that reported an excess of births during January, February, and March in a group of Danish schizophrenic patients with a family history of schizophrenia, an outcome that reinforced their view that viral infections might be etiologically significant for adult schizophrenia (Machon et al. 1983). Moreover, a series of investigations following the 1953 and 1957 influenza epidemics (Coffey and Jessop 1955, 1959; Hakosalo and Saxen 1971) had noted an increased frequency of neural tube defects among exposed offspring, supporting the assertion that in utero exposure to influenza could cause central nervous system disorder (see Chapter 5, this volume).

These investigators therefore undertook the first investigation of the prenatal influenza hypothesis of schizophrenia. They reported that the risk of schizophrenia was increased by about 50% for Finnish individuals exposed to the 1957 A2 influenza epidemic during their second trimester of gestation (Mednick et al. 1988). This first report led to a flurry of attempts at replication. To date, at least 15 studies have been performed in several different countries and in both hemispheres; these studies have examined influenza epidemics in a single year (usually 1957) as well as the annually varying prevalence of influenza infection over several decades. Ten of the studies reported a positive association between prenatal influenza exposure and schizophrenia (Adams et al. 1993 [the 1957 pandemic]; Barr et al. 1990; Fahy et al. 1993; Kunugi et al. 1995; McGrath et al. 1994; Mednick et al. 1988; O'Callaghan et al. 1991b; Sham et al. 1992; Takei et al. 1994a, 1994b), while six either produced equivocal results (Adams et al. 1993 [longitudinal analysis]; Kendell and Kemp 1989; Takei et al. 1995b) or found no association (Erlenmeyer-Kimling et al. 1994; Selten and Sleats 1994; Susser et al. 1994; Torrey et al. 1991) (Table 4–1). These studies were not necessarily independent tests of the prenatal influenza/schizophrenia hypothesis, since some data were overlapping; in particular, the same data source was used by both Selten and Sleats (1994) and Susser et al. (1994).

Our research group's results from England and Wales serve to illustrate the positive associations that have been reported (O'Callaghan et al. 1991b). The 1957 influenza epidemic reached its peak (as measured by both claims for sickness benefit and contemporaneous serological data) in England in late September and early October. We compared the number of schizophrenic births in the months following this peak with the number of births in the corresponding months of the 2 previous years and the 2 subsequent years. Five months after the epidemic, there was an 88% increase in

Table 4–1. Studies of schizophrenia and influenza epidemics

Author	Location	Result
Mednick et al. 1988	Finland	2nd-trimester exposure associated with increased risk
Kendell and Kemp 1989	Scotland	Association between 6th-month exposure and increased risk among females in Edinburgh but not in Scotland overall
Barr et al. 1990	Denmark	6th-month exposure associated with increased risk over 40 years
O'Callaghan et al. 1991b	England/Wales	5th-month exposure associated with increased risk, more marked in females
Kunugi et al. 1992	Tokyo, Japan	4th-month exposure associated with increased risk
Sham et al. 1992	England/Wales	6th-/7th-month exposure associated with increased risk over 22 years
Torrey et al. 1992	10 states, USA	No significant association
Adams et al. 1993	Scotland	4th-month exposure associated with increased risk in females
	England/Wales	4th-month exposure associated with increased risk
	Denmark	6th-month exposure associated with increased risk
Fahy et al. 1993	England	5th-month exposure associated with increased risk, more marked in females (Afro-Caribbeans)
McGrath et al. 1994	Queensland, Australia	5th-month exposure associated with increased risk, mainly females
Selten and Sleats 1994	Holland	No significant association

(continued)

Table 4–1.   Studies of schizophrenia and influenza epidemics
(continued)

Author	Location	Result
Susser et al. 1994	Holland	No significant association
Takei et al. 1994a	England/Wales	5th-month exposure associated with increased risk in females over 28 years
Takei et al. 1994b	Denmark	6th-month exposure associated with increased risk over 56 years
Takei et al. 1995a	Holland	Association between "typical" schizophrenia and exposure 3 months before birth

the number of births of individuals destined to develop schizophrenia. The temporal relationship between gestational influenza exposure and birth has been relatively consistent in the positive studies reported so far, and suggests that the 4th through 7th months of gestation present a window of opportunity that allows the influenza virus to have a damaging effect. When we compared the months of birth of schizophrenic patients in England and Wales in high- and low-influenza years, we found that the years that had more influenza deaths were also the years with a greater spring excess of schizophrenic births. Using a Poisson regression model, we estimated that up to 2% of all cases of schizophrenia, and 4% of cases of schizophrenia in patients born in late winter and spring, might be attributable to influenza (Sham et al. 1992). Even for very large influenza epidemics, our model predicted an increased risk of only 10%–20%, suggesting that the 88% increase in births of future schizophrenic patients we reported for the 1957 epidemic would be an uncommon occurrence. Crow (1995) has criticized this seemingly different effect size, but his criticism may specifically relate to a failure to differentiate between *risk difference percentage* (the proportion of cases in an exposed group that are attributed to the exposure) and *population-attributable risk fraction* (the proportion of all cases in a study population that are attributed to the exposure) (Takei et al. 1995a). Thus, one may reasonably conclude that influenza may account for almost half of all schizophrenia cases among the population exposed to the 1957 epidemic, *not* among the population as a whole or among those exposed to other influenza epidemics.

Reports of an association between schizophrenia and prenatal influenza exposure have been criticized on several grounds. The short duration of the excess of births, the lack of uniformity in the results (Crow and Done 1992) and the negative U.S. study (Torrey et al. 1992), the inconsistency between studies in the timing of the excess (Crow 1994), the complexity of the statistical models used in the analyses (Crow 1994), and the testing of multiple months (Curtis 1992) have all been reasonably cited as grounds for caution. On the other hand, such criticisms do not explain the many positive associations reported for the 4th through 7th months of gestation by several independent research groups working in different countries—and, indeed, in different hemispheres. It may be that prenatal influenza does increase the risk of schizophrenia but that the overall effect size is small and is thus undetectable in some studies. Furthermore, contrary to some suggestions (Crow 1994), it may be that sophisticated statistical methods are sometimes necessary to separate out the true effect of gestational influenza exposure from confounders and random fluctuations. Thus, Takei and colleagues (1995b) have promoted the use of Poisson regression analysis, citing the growing use of this technique in other fields of medicine. Kuhn and associates (1994), for example, used this technique to control for both time trends and seasonality factors when evaluating the effect of a prevention program on longitudinal rates for child injury, and claimed that Poisson regression provides a versatile analytical method for quantifying the time trends of relatively discrete outcomes (Kuhn et al. 1994).

Studies of individuals rather than populations would further test the prenatal influenza/schizophrenia hypothesis, and some such studies have been performed (Table 4–2). The first cohort study was reported by Crow and colleagues (1991) and was based on the British National Child Development Survey (NCDS) of 1958,

Table 4–2. Cohort and case–control studies of maternal influenza and schizophrenia

Author	Location	Design	Result
Crow et al. 1991	England	Cohort	No significant association
Cannon et al. 1994	Ireland	Cohort	No significant association
Stober et al. 1992	Germany	Case–control	2nd-trimester exposure associated with schizophrenia
Mednick et al. 1994	Finland	Case–control	2nd-trimester exposure associated with schizophrenia
Wright et al. 1995b	England	Case–control	2nd-trimester exposure associated with schizophrenia

which, by chance, was initiated 5 months after the influenza epidemic of 1957. It was found that children whose mothers reported influenza during the second trimester of gestation were no more likely than control children to develop schizophrenia. Similarly, Cannon and co-workers (1996) followed a cohort of Irish children born after the 1957 influenza epidemic who were originally studied for neural tube defects (Coffey and Jessop 1955, 1959), and they found no association between maternal influenza during pregnancy and later schizophrenia in the offspring. The NCDS results have been questioned, both on the grounds that the study had limited power to detect the proposed association and because nonstandard statistical methods were used (Takei et al. 1995b); similar criticisms can be made of the study by Cannon et al. (1996).

In contrast, results supporting the hypothesized schizophrenia–prenatal influenza association have been reported by three other case–control studies. Stober and colleagues (1992) studied 55 patients with chronic schizophrenia and 20 control subjects and found that although there was no significant difference in the overall rate of maternal infections during pregnancy (24% vs. 20%), significantly more of the infections reported by the mothers of schizophrenia patients occurred during the second trimester (9 of 13 infections). Mednick and associates (1994) reviewed the contemporaneous antenatal records of the mothers of schizophrenic patients born after the 1957 influenza epidemic in Helsinki, Finland, and found that 86.7% (13 of 15) of those exposed to the epidemic during the second trimester had influenza symptoms recorded by midwives in their medical notes, compared with only 20% (2 of 10) of those exposed to the epidemic during the first or third trimesters of pregnancy. Our research group undertook a within-subjects controlled study and found that the mothers of 121 schizophrenic patients reported a significant excess of influenza during the second trimester of their offsprings' gestations, compared with the combined first and third trimesters (11.6% vs. 1.7%; odds ratio [OR] = 7.79, 95% confidence interval [CI] = 1.63–50.81, P = .002). Furthermore, mothers who reported second-trimester influenza had a significantly increased risk of obstetric complications during pregnancy (OR = 4.84, 95% CI = 1.31–19.70, P = .011), and the schizophrenic offspring of these mothers weighed an average of 210 grams less at birth than the offspring whose mothers had not suffered second-trimester influenza (Wright et al. 1995b).

Takei and Murray (1994) have pointed out the low statistical power of cohort studies for detecting risk factors for a rare disease. Given that schizophrenia affects between 0.5% and 1% of the population, several thousand individuals would need to be followed longitudinally in order to obtain even a relatively small number of cases. Although O'Callaghan and colleagues (1991b) have estimated that relative risks as high as 2 or 3 could not be excluded on the basis of the NCDS data, cohort studies to date lend no support to the hypothesized association between schizophrenia and prenatal influenza. However, the three retrospective case–control studies do offer such support, and their results are both remarkably consistent and in keeping with those population studies that identify maximum risk with the second trimester. These studies may be subject to bias due to selective recall of adverse events during gestations of offspring who later developed schizophrenia. Nonetheless, as regards our own study, it is difficult to see how any systematic recall bias could account for either the excess of infections reported in the second trimester or the associations between infections and both obstetric complications and reduction in mean birthweight (Wright et al. 1995b).

Could Maternal Influenza Perturb Fetal Neurodevelopment?

If we accept that prenatal influenza exposure and adult schizophrenia may be associated and that a proportion of schizophrenia cases involve neuropathology suggestive of a neurodevelopmental etiology, we must next consider mechanisms by which maternal influenza could impair fetal neurodevelopment and set the stage for schizophrenia two or three decades later. The influenza virus could perturb fetal neurodevelopment either by direct infection of the fetal brain or by one of several indirect means.

Influenza is a systemic disease. Although its extrarespiratory symptoms can include fever, myalgia, arthralgia, encephalitis, and myocarditis, these are mediated not by a viremia (Murphy and Webster 1990) but rather by soluble components of the host's immune response to influenza infection such as antibodies and cytokines (Cohen and Lisak 1987). Cases of transplacental fetal influenza infection have been reported, but in even the most convincing of these, infection occurred toward the end of gestation, and isolation of influenza virus from amniotic fluid raises the possibility of a transcervical route of spread (McGregor et al. 1984; Yawn et al. 1971). Furthermore, intracardiac inoculation with enormous quantities of virus is necessary in order to achieve transplacental transfer of influenza virus in an animal model (Rushton et al. 1983). For this reason, the influenza virus is usually confined to the epithelial cells of the maternal respiratory tract; thus, any deleterious effect on the fetus may more likely involve an indirect mechanism such as fever, hypoxia, acid-base imbalance, anti-influenza medications, or nutritional deficiency (see Chapter 5, this volume).

However, these indirect effects are not specific to any particular virus, and influenza represents the only virus in which associations with schizophrenia have been independently replicated. We have therefore postulated that some factor derived from the maternal immune system may mediate the effects of influenza virus in the developing fetal brain in utero. The teratogenic antibody hypothesis thus suggests that some proportion of schizophrenia cases may represent an autoimmune disease by proxy. According to our hypothesis, antibodies of maternal origin are elicited in immunogenetically predisposed women by the influenza virus, cross the placenta and the immature fetal blood–brain barrier during the second trimester of gestation, and disrupt fetal neurodevelopment by cross-reacting with brain antigens via molecular mimicry (Laing et al. 1995; Wright and Murray 1993; Wright et al. 1993).

Is such a process biologically plausible? Induction of antibodies to a brain-specific protein has been reported after inoculation of rabbits with influenza virus (Laing et al. 1989), and Knight (1991) has argued that immunological damage to the fetus may be most likely in women who mount a particularly effective immune response and who therefore have the mildest clinical symptoms. Indeed, this was suggested as a possible explanation of the negative findings by Crow and colleagues (1991). One direct test of the hypothesis that prenatal influenza exposure could cause neuropathological lesions has been performed. Cotter and co-workers (1995) exposed mice to influenza A in utero and conducted neuropathological studies of the animals' brains 21 days after birth. They found no overall evidence that prenatal influenza exposure increased hippocampal pyramidal cell disarray in exposed mice compared with controls; however, there was a modest effect for mice exposed on day 13 of gestation, the approximate murine equivalent of the second trimester of gestation in humans.

Can the Teratogenic Antibody Hypothesis Be Tested?

The cardinal features of the teratogenic antibody hypothesis are influenza exposure during the second trimester of gestation and maternal immunogenetic predisposition to elaborate the offending antibody. In addition, there may be a genetic factor that determines fetal susceptibility to the postulated teratogen. We have tested our hypothesis by investigating 1) maternal and proband immunogenes, 2) maternal recall of influenza during the proband's gestation and any association with clinical features suggestive of neurodevelopmental anomaly, and 3) antibrain antibody activity in sera from probands, their mothers, and control subjects. In the following paragraphs we discuss our findings and the tentative conclusions that we draw from them.

Maternal and Proband Immunogenes

In humans, the human leukocyte antigens (HLA) A1, A2, and A3 are important in the elimination of influenza virus by killer lymphocytes (DiBrino et al. 1993; Morrison et al. 1992). Thus, one approach toward validating our hypothesis is to search for an unusual distribution of HLA A1, A2, and A3 in the mothers of schizophrenic patients. (We therefore examined this in mothers of 121 schizophrenic offspring but found no unusual distribution of these antigens.)

Another approach is to examine the relationship between schizophrenia and the alleles encoding HLA DR4 at the HLA DRB1 locus on the short arm of chromosome 6. A negative association has been consistently demonstrated between schizophrenia and rheumatoid arthritis (Eaton et al. 1992), a systemic autoimmune disease associated with HLA DR4 (Tsuji et al. 1992). We therefore tested the hypothesis that schizophrenia may be negatively associated with HLA DR4 and found that 25 of 93 schizophrenic subjects, as compared with 79 of 177 control subjects, were DR4 positive (Wright et al. 1996a). To further explore this finding, we examined the frequency distribution of HLA DR4 in an unrelated cohort of 91 women who had given birth to offspring who subsequently developed schizophrenia; they exhibited a deficiency of DR4 of similar magnitude (see Table 4–3) (Wright et al. 1996a). Perhaps, therefore, HLA DR4 exerts a protective role against schizophrenia (Wright et al. 1996a). In addition, we found an excess of insulin-dependent diabetes mellitus in the first-degree relatives of schizophrenic patients compared with control subjects, and we in-

Table 4–3. Proportion of schizophrenic patients, mothers of schizophrenic patients, and control subjects positive for human leukocyte antigen (HLA) DR4

HLA antigen tested	Sample	Finding	Statistical values
DR4	93 schizophrenic patients 177 control subjects	25 schizophrenic patients (26.9%) 79 control subjects (44.6%)	OR = 0.46, 95% CI = 0.25–0.81, $\chi^2 = 8.11, P = .004$
DR4[a]	91 mothers of schizophrenic probands	23 mothers (25.3%)	OR = 0.42 95% CI = 0.23–0.76 $\chi^2 = 9.55, P = .002$

Note. CI = confidence interval; OR = odds ratio.
[a] The schizophrenic subjects and mothers of schizophrenic subjects were unrelated to each other (i.e., the 93 probands were not the offspring of the 91 mothers, and both samples were collected independently).
Source. Wright et al. 1995b.

terpret this as further evidence of genetic predisposition to autoimmunity in the pedigrees of some schizophrenic patients (Wright et al. 1996b), although there may be other explanations. Therefore, while not definitive, these findings go some way toward implicating an autoimmune mechanism in the etiology of schizophrenia.

Maternal Recall of Influenza During the Proband's Gestation

The results of our structured interviews with the mothers of 121 schizophrenic patients were described earlier in this chapter. Briefly, these women recalled a significant excess of influenza during the second trimester, compared with the combined first and third trimesters, of their offsprings' gestations (11.6% vs. 1.7%, $P = .002$), and there was also a significant association between second-trimester influenza and obstetric complications during pregnancy (OR = 4.84, 95% CI = 1.31–19.70, $P = .011$) (Wright et al. 1995b).

Antibrain Antibody Activity in Sera From Probands

As previously discussed, it has been shown that influenza viruses are capable of eliciting autoantibodies in experimental animals, and autoantibodies against a 37-kilodalton (kD) brain protein have been detected in rabbits immunized with certain influenza A viruses (Laing et al. 1989). We have preliminary evidence that the mothers of schizophrenic patients have higher titers of antibodies to an 87–88-kD antigen derived from rat brain than do control subjects, with their schizophrenic offspring exhibiting levels intermediate between those of mothers and control subjects (Jameel 1993). Thus, it may be that maternal and/or proband antibrain antibodies are responsible, in whole or part, for some cases of schizophrenia. It is therefore of interest that Kilidireas and colleagues (1992) have demonstrated a significantly increased occurrence of the antibody to the P1 mitochondrial heat shock protein (hsp60) in individuals with schizophrenia compared with control subjects; infection is known to induce formation of this autoantibody (see Chapter 9, this volume).

Finally, while HLA studies in schizophrenia have been inconsistent and inconclusive overall, a weakly positive association between paranoid schizophrenia and HLA A9 has been found in seven of nine studies (McGuffin and Sturt 1986; Wright et al. 1993). We also found an excess of A9 in our sample, and this was almost wholly composed of the A24 subspecificity of A9 (25.0% vs. 14.2%, OR = 2.02, 95% CI = 0.98–4.15, P = .04) (Wright et al. 1995a). Although neither HLA A9 nor HLA A24 has been specifically implicated in modulation of the immune response to influenza, these findings may represent further evidence of an immune abnormality in schizophrenia.

What Next?

Kirch (1993) have highlighted the interaction between infectious agents and host immune response and the effect of this interaction on the developing brain as areas of high priority for future research. The results from our group and others suggest that prenatal influenza exposure may account for a portion of schizophrenia cases. Because only a small number of influenza-exposed pregnancies give rise to schizophrenia, however, we propose that an interaction between genetic predisposition and influenza infection is necessary. In schizophrenic probands and their mothers, we have found preliminary evidence of immunogenetic abnormalities, some of which might account for an abnormal immune response to influenza infection, with resultant damage to the developing fetal brain. While these findings are far from conclusive, the role of immune, genetic, and infectious factors in the etiopathogenesis of schizophrenia is substantially increasing in importance. Therefore, like Kirch, we believe that it is time to make a concerted effort to unravel the immunology and immunogenetics of schizophrenia.

References

Adams W, Kendell RE, Hare EH, et al: Epidemiological evidence that maternal influenza contributes to the aetiology of schizophrenia: an analysis of Scottish, English and Danish data. Br J Psychiatry 163:522–534, 1993

Barr CE, Mednick SA, Munk-Jorgensen P: Exposure to influenza epidemics during gestation and adult schizophrenia: a 40-year study. Arch Gen Psychiatry 47:869–874, 1990

Bellodi L, Bussolini C, Scorza-Smeraldi S, et al: Family study of schizophrenia: exploratory analysis of relevant factors. Schizophr Bull 12:120–128, 1986

Boyd JH, Pulver AE, Stewart W: Season of birth: schizophrenia and bipolar disorder. Schizophr Bull 12:173–186, 1986

Bradbury TN, Miller GA: Season of birth in schizophrenia: a review of evidence, methodology, and etiology. Psychol Bull 98:569–594, 1985

Buck C, Simpson H: Season of birth among the sibs of schizophrenics. Br J Psychiatry 132:358–360, 1978

Cannon M, Cotter D, Coffey VP, et al: Prenatal exposure to the 1957 influenza epidemic and adult schizophrenia: a follow-up study. Br J Psychiatry 168:368–371, 1996

Coffey VP, Jessop WJE: Congenital abnormalities—6th series. Ir J Med Sci 349:30–46, 1955

Coffey VP, Jessop WJE: Maternal influenza and congenital deformities: a prospective study. Lancet 2:935–938, 1959

Cohen JA, Lisak RP: Acute disseminated encephalomyelitis, in Clinical Neuroimmunology. Edited by Aarli JA, Behan WMH, Behan PO. Oxford, England, Blackwell Scientific, 1987

Cotter D, Farrell M, Takei N, et al: Does prenatal exposure to influenza in mice induce pyramidal disarray in the hippocampus? Schizophr Res 16:233–241, 1995

Crow TJ: A re-evaluation of the viral hypothesis: is psychosis the result of retroviral integration at a site close to the cerebral dominance gene? Br J Psychiatry 145:243–253, 1984

Crow TJ: Prenatal influenza as a cause of schizophrenia: there are inconsistencies and contradictions in the evidence. Br J Psychiatry 164:588–592, 1994

Crow TJ: Comments on Takei et al.: Prenatal exposure to influenza epidemics and the risk of mental retardation (letter). Eur Arch Psychiatry Clin Neurosci 245:1–2, 1995

Crow TJ, Done DJ: Prenatal exposure to influenza does not cause schizophrenia. Br J Psychiatry 161:390–393, 1992

Crow TJ, Done DJ, Johnstone EC: Schizophrenia and influenza. Lancet 338:116–117, 1991

Curtis D: Schizophrenia following prenatal exposure to influenza epidemics between 1939 and 1960. Br J Psychiatry 161:712–713, 1992

Dalen P: Season of birth: a study of schizophrenia and other mental disorders. Amsterdam, North Holland, 1975

DiBrino M, Tsuchida T, Turner R, et al: HLA A1 and HLA A3 T-cell epitopes derived from influenza virus proteins predicted from peptide binding motifs. J Immunol 11:5930–5935, 1993

Eaton WW, Hayward C, Ram R: Schizophrenia and rheumatoid arthritis: a review. Schizophr Res 6:181–192, 1992

Erlenmeyer-Kimling L, Folnegovic Z, Hrabak-Zerjavic Boracic B, et al: Schizophrenia and prenatal exposure to the 1957 A2 influenza epidemic in Croatia. Am J Psychiatry 151:1496–1498, 1994

Fahy TA, Jones PB, Sham PC: Schizophrenia in Afro-Caribbeans in the UK following prenatal exposure to the 1957 A2 influenza epidemic. Schizophr Res 6:98–99, 1993

Gibbs CJ, Gajdusek DC: Neurologic diseases of man with slow virus etiology, in Membranes and Viruses in Immunopathology. Edited by Day SB, Good RA. New York, Academic Press, 1972, pp 397–409

Goldstein JM: Gender and schizophrenia: a summary of findings. Schizophrenia Monitor 2:1–4, 1992

Gordon CT, Frazier JA, McKenna K, et al: Childhood-onset schizophrenia: an NIMH study in process. Schizophr Bull 20:697–712, 1994

Gosline HI: Newer conception of dementia praecox based on unrecognised work. J Lab Clin Med 2:691–698, 1917

Gosline HI: The role of tuberculosis in dementia praecox. J Lab Clin Med 4:186–192, 1919

Gottesman II: Schizophrenia Genesis: The Origins of Madness. New York, Freeman, 1991

Gottesman II, Shields J: Schizophrenia: The Epigenetic Puzzle. Cambridge, England, Cambridge University Press, 1982

Hakosalo JK, Saxen L: Influenza epidemic and congenital defects. Lancet 2:1346–1347, 1971

Hare EH: The season of birth of siblings of psychiatric patients. Br J Psychiatry 129:49–54, 1976

Hare EH, Price JS, Slater E: Schizophrenia and season of birth. Br J Psychiatry 120:125–126, 1972

Hare EH, Price JS, Slater E: Mental disorder and season of birth: a national survey compared with the general population. Br J Psychiatry 152:460–465, 1974

Jameel SY: Studies of virus induced autoimmunity to brain antigens in schizophrenia. B Med Sci thesis, University of Nottingham, England, 1993

Jones IH, Frei D: Seasonal births in schizophrenia: a Southern Hemisphere study using matched parts. Acta Psychiatr Scand 59:164–172, 1979

Kendell RE, Kemp IW: Maternal influenza in the aetiology of schizophrenia. Arch Gen Psychiatry 46:878–882, 1989

Kendler KS: Overview: a current perspective on twin studies of schizophrenia. Am J Psychiatry 140:1413–1420, 1983

Kilidireas K, Latov N, Strauss DH, et al: Antibodies to the human 60 kDa heat-shock protein in patients with schizophrenia. Lancet 340:569–572, 1992

Kirch DG: Infection and autoimmunity as aetiological factors in schizophrenia: a review and reappraisal. Schizophr Bull 19:355–370, 1993

Knight JG: Schizophrenia and influenza. Lancet 338:390–392, 1991

Kraepelin E: Dementia Praecox and Paraphrenia. Translated by Barclay RM. Edinburgh, Scotland, E&S Livingstone, 1919

Kuhn L, Davidson LL, Durkin MS: Use of Poisson regression and time series analysis for detecting changes over time in rates of child injury following a prevention programme. Am J Epidemiol 140:943–955, 1994

Kunugi H, Nanko S, Takei N: Influenza and schizophrenia in Japan. Br J Psychiatry 161:274–275, 1992

Kunugi H, Nanko S, Takei N, et al: Schizophrenia following in utero exposure to the 1957 influenza epidemics in Japan. Am J Psychiatry 152: 450–452, 1995

Laing P, Knight JG, Hill JM, et al: Influenza viruses induce autoantibodies to a brain specific 37 kDa protein in rabbit. Proc Natl Acad Sci U S A 86:1998–2002, 1989

Laing P, Knight JG, Wright P, et al: Disruption of fetal development by maternal antibodies as an etiological factor in schizophrenia, in Neural Development in Schizophrenia: Theory and Research. Edited by Mednick SA, Hollister JM. New York, Plenum, 1995, pp 215–246

Lewis MS, Griffin TA: An explanation for the season of birth effect in schizophrenia and certain other diseases. Psychol Bull 89:589–596, 1981

Lewis SW: Congenital risk factors for schizophrenia. Psychol Med 19:5–13, 1989

Lewis SW, Murray RM: Obstetric complications, neurodevelopmental deviance, and risk of schizophrenia. J Psychiatr Res 21:413–421, 1987

Libikova H, Breir S, Kosikova M, et al: Assay of interferon and viral antibodies in the cerebrospinal fluid in clinical neurology and psychiatry. Acta Biologica Medica Germanica 38:879–893, 1979

Machon RA, Mednick SA, Schulsinger F: The interaction of seasonality, place of birth, genetic risk and subsequent schizophrenia in a high risk sample. Br J Psychiatry 143:383–388, 1983

McGrath JJ, Pemberton M, Welham JL, et al: Schizophrenia and the influenza epidemics of 1954, 1957 and 1959: a Southern Hemisphere study. Schizophr Res 14:1–8, 1994

McGregor JA, Burns JC, Levin MJ, et al: Transplacental passage of influenza A Bangkok (H3N2) mimicking amniotic fluid infection syndrome. Am J Obstet Gynecol 149:856–863, 1984

McGuffin P, Sturt E: Genetic markers in schizophrenia. Hum Hered 36: 65–88, 1986

McGuffin P, Asherson P, Owen M, et al: The strength of the genetic effect: is there room for an environmental influence in the aetiology of schizophrenia? Br J Psychiatry 164:593–599, 1994

McGuffin P, Owen MJ, Farmer AE: Genetic basis of schizophrenia. Lancet 346:678–682, 1995

McGuire PK, Jones P, Harvey I, et al: Cannabis and acute psychosis. Schizophr Res 13:161–168, 1994

McNeil TF, Kaij L, Dzierzykray-Rogalska M: Season of birth among siblings of schizophrenics. Acta Psychiatr Scand 54:267–274, 1976

Mednick SA, Machon RA, Huttunen MO, et al: Adult schizophrenia following prenatal exposure to an influenza epidemic. Arch Gen Psychiatry 45:189–192, 1988

Mednick SA, Huttunen MO, Machon RA: Prenatal influenza infections and adult schizophrenia. Schizophr Bull 20:263–267, 1994

Menninger KA: The schizophrenic syndromes as a product of acute infectious disease. Archives of Neurology and Psychiatry 20:464–481, 1928

Morrison J, Elvin J, Latron F, et al: Identification of the nonamer peptide from influenza A matrix protein and the role of pockets of HLA A2 in its recognition by cytotoxic T lymphocytes. Eur J Immunol 22:903–907, 1992

Murphy BR, Webster RG: Orthomyxoviruses, in Virology, 2nd Edition. Edited by Fields BN, Knipe DM. New York, Raven, 1990, pp 1091–1152

O'Callaghan E, Gibson T, Colohan HA, et al: Season of birth in schizophrenia: evidence for confinement of an excess of winter births to patients without a family history of mental disorder. Br J Psychiatry 158:764–769, 1991a

O'Callaghan E, Sham PC, Takei N, et al: Schizophrenia after prenatal exposure to 1957 A2 influenza epidemic. Lancet 337:1248–1250, 1991b

Pallast EG, Jongbloet PH, Straatman HM, et al: Excess seasonality of births among patients with schizophrenia and seasonal ovopathy. Schizophr Bull 20:269–276, 1994

Parker G, Neilson M: Mental disorder and season of birth: a Southern Hemisphere study. Br J Psychiatry 129:355–361, 1976

Pulver AE, Liang KY, Wolyniec PS, et al: Season of birth among siblings of schizophrenic patients. Br J Psychiatry 160:71–75, 1992

Rao DC, Morton NE, Gottesman II, et al: Path analysis of qualitative data on pairs of relatives: application to schizophrenia. Hum Hered 31:325–333, 1981

Rushton DI, Collie MH, Sweet C, et al: The effects of maternal influenza viraemia in late gestation on the conceptus of the pregnant ferret. J Pathol 140:181–189, 1983

Selten JPCJ, Sleats JPJ: Evidence against maternal influenza as a risk factor for schizophrenia. Br J Psychiatry 164:674–676, 1994

Sham PC, O'Callaghan E, Takei N, et al: Schizophrenia following prenatal exposure to influenza epidemics between 1939 and 1960. Br J Psychiatry 160:461–466, 1992

Sham PC, Jones P, Russell A, et al: Age at onset, sex and familial psychiatric morbidity in schizophrenia: Camberwell collaborative psychosis study. Br J Psychiatry 165:466–473, 1994

Sierra-Honigmann AM, Carbone KM, Yolken RH: Polymerase chain reaction (PCR) search for viral nucleic acid sequences in schizophrenia. Br J Psychiatry 166:55–60, 1995

Skliar N: Psychoses in infectious diseases, especially typhus and recurrent fevers. Monatschrier Psychiatrie Neurologique 2:21–27, 1922

Stober G, Franzek E, Beckmann J: The role of maternal infectious diseases during pregnancy in the aetiology of schizophrenia in offspring. European Psychiatry 7:147–152, 1992

Susser E, Lin SP, Brown AS, et al: No relation between risk of schizophrenia and prenatal exposure to influenza in Holland. Am J Psychiatry 151:922–924, 1994

Takei N, Murray RM: Prenatal influenza and schizophrenia. Br J Psychiatry 165:833–834, 1994

Takei N, Mortensen MD, Klaening U, et al: Relationship between in utero exposure to influenza epidemics and risk of schizophrenia in Denmark (letter). Schizophr Res 11:95, 1994a

Takei N, Sham PC, O'Callaghan E, et al: Prenatal exposure to influenza and the development of schizophrenia: is the effect confined to females? Am J Psychiatry 151:117–119, 1994b

Takei N, Van Os J, Murray RM: Maternal exposure to influenza and risk of schizophrenia: a 22-year study from The Netherlands. J Psychiatr Res 29:435–445, 1995a

Takei N, Murray RM, Sham P, et al: Reply to comments on Takei et al.: Prenatal exposure to influenza epidemics and the risk of mental retardation (letter). Eur Arch Psychiatry Clin Neurosci 245:4–7, 1995b

Torrey EF: Slow and latent viruses in schizophrenia. Lancet 2:22–24, 1973

Torrey EF: Stalking the schizovirus. Schizophr Res 14:223–229, 1988

Torrey EF, Yolken RH, Winfrey CJ: Cytomegalovirus antibody in cerebrospinal fluid of schizophrenic patients detected by enzyme immunoassay. Science 216:892–893, 1982

Torrey EF, Bowler AE, Rawlings R: An influenza epidemic and the seasonality of schizophrenic births, in Psychiatry and Biological Factors. Edited by Kurstat K. New York, Plenum, 1991, pp 106–116

Torrey EF, Bowler AE, Rawlings R: Schizophrenia and the 1957 influenza epidemic. Schizophr Res 6:100–107, 1992

Tsuji K, Aizawa M, Sasazuki T (eds): Proceedings of the Eleventh International Histocompatibility Workshop and Conference, Held in Yokohama, Japan, 6–13 November 1991. Oxford, England, Oxford University Press, 1992

Watson CG, Kucala T, Tilleskjor C, et al: Schizophrenic birth seasonality in relation to the incidence of infectious diseases and temperature extremes. Arch Gen Psychiatry 41:85–90, 1984

Welham JL, Pemberton MR, McGrath JJ: Schizophrenia: do seasonal birth rates vary between hemispheres? Schizophr Res 9:142–143, 1993

Wolyniec PS, Pulver AE, McGrath JA, et al: Schizophrenia: gender and familial risk. J Psychiatric Res 26:17–27, 1992

Wrede G, Mednick SA, Huttunen MO, et al: Pregnancy and delivery complications in the births of an unselected series of Finnish children with schizophrenic mothers. Acta Psychiatr Scand 62:369–381, 1980

Wright P, Murray RM: Prenatal influenza, immunogenes and schizophrenia, in The Neurodevelopmental Basis of Schizophrenia. Edited by Waddington JL, Buckley PF. Austin, TX, RG Landes, 1995, pp 43–59

Wright P, Gill M, Murray RM: Schizophrenia: genetics and the maternal immune response to viral infection. Am J Med Genet 48:40–46, 1993

Wright P, Donaldson PT, Curtis VA, et al: Immunogenetic markers in schizophrenia: HLA A9 revisited (abstract). Schizophr Res 15:50, 1995a

Wright P, Rifkin L, Takei N, et al: Maternal influenza, obstetric complications and schizophrenia. Am J Psychiatry 152:1714–1720, 1995b

Wright P, Donaldson PT, Underhill JA, et al: Genetic association of the HLA DRB1 locus on chromosome 6p21.3 with schizophrenia. Am J Psychiatry 153:1530–1533, 1996a

Wright P, Sham PC, Gilvarry CM, et al: Autoimmune diseases in the pedigrees of schizophrenic and control subjects. Schizophr Res 20:261–267, 1996b

Yawn DH, Pyeatte JC, Joseph JM, et al: Transplacental transfer of influenza virus. JAMA 1216:1022–1023, 1971

Yolken RH, Petric M, Collett M, et al: Pestivirus infection in identical twins discordant for schizophrenia (letter). Schizophr Res 9:231, 1993

Chapter 5

Plausibility of Prenatal Rubella, Influenza, and Other Viral Infections as Risk Factors for Schizophrenia

Alan S. Brown, M.D., and Ezra S. Susser, M.D., Dr.P.H.

As reviewed by Wright and colleagues in Chapter 4, evidence of associations between gestational exposure to viral epidemics and adult schizophrenia suggests that prenatal viral exposure may play an etiological role in schizophrenia (Barr et al. 1990; Kunugi et al. 1995; Mednick et al. 1988; O'Callaghan et al. 1991, 1994; Sham et al. 1992; Torrey et al. 1988; Watson et al. 1984). These findings provide further support for the neurodevelopmental hypothesis of schizophrenia, which asserts that a proportion of schizophrenia cases result from disruptions in early brain development (Chapter 1, this volume).

We shall examine the neurobiological plausibility of prenatal infections, especially rubella and influenza, as risk factors for schizophrenia. In this chapter, we discuss the following: 1) concordance in the developmental pathology between prenatal viral infection and schizophrenia; 2) known viral causes of congenital central nervous system (CNS) malformations; 3) epidemiological and pathogenic evidence for and against influenza infection as a cause of CNS malformations; and 4) potential causal pathways of prenatal influenza as a cause of schizophrenia. We shall infer that the findings argue against a simple causal model and suggest instead the possibility of a complex interplay between a viral exposure and other mediating or interacting factors.

Concordance in Developmental Pathology Between Prenatal Viral Infection and Schizophrenia

Evidence from several studies points to a concordance between the developmental pathology produced by viral infection and the abnormalities found in schizophrenia. With respect to neuropathology, both individuals exposed to prenatal viral infections such as herpes simplex and individuals with schizophrenia (Waddington 1993) have ventriculomegaly and temporolimbic abnormalities. Higher rates of dermatoglyphic disturbances have also been demonstrated both in persons prenatally exposed to rubella (Achs et al. 1966; Purvis-Smith and Menser 1973) and cytomegalovirus (Purvis-Smith et al. 1972) and in patients with schizophrenia (Green et al. 1989; O'Callaghan et al. 1991). Delayed psychomotor and neuromotor development and childhood behavioral disturbances have been found in both individuals exposed in utero to viral infection (Chess et al. 1971; Ho 1991; Whitley and Stagno 1991) and individuals destined to develop schizophrenia (Fish et al. 1992; Jones et al. 1994; E. F. Walker et al. 1994). Finally, the early to midgestational timing of occurrence of the developmental pathology in many congenital infections is proposed to be similar to the timing of the putative insult in neurodevelopmental schizophrenia (Waddington 1993; Whitley and Stagno 1991).

Known Viral Causes of CNS Malformations

A review of known viral causes of CNS malformations of neuroviruses is a logical starting point in the search for neurodevelopmental viral causes of schizophrenia. In this light, we present examples of viruses that affect CNS development and pathogenic mechanisms by which viruses disrupt CNS development.

Research over the past 50 years has established that many viral agents cause congenital brain disorders. Among the best known of the viral teratogens are rubella, cytomegalovirus, and herpes simplex virus. We have selected these three viral agents for focus here because they each illustrate specific and important conceptual features that need to be considered in developing a plausible and coherent theory of prenatal viral infection as a cause of schizophrenia.

Rubella

As the most frequently cited viral cause of congenital anomalies, rubella provides a model for infectious teratogenic effects in early gestation. The congenital rubella syndrome was first described by Sir Norman Gregg, who noted a possible causal association between maternal rubella infection during gestation and congenital cataracts in offspring (Gregg 1942; Gregg et al. 1945). Studies of rubella have established that a first-trimester infection, following transmission from mother to fetus via the placenta (Whitley and Stagno 1991), can indeed impair fetal development and result in prominent CNS congenital malformations (Desmond et al. 1967, 1969). In addition, a variety of behavioral disorders found in individuals destined to develop schizophrenia, including separation anxiety, disruptiveness, rituals, and impaired social relations, have been reported in children of mothers infected with rubella during pregnancy (Chess et al. 1971). Moreover, the pattern of brain dysmorphology in patients with schizophrenia is similar to that in individuals with congenital rubella accompanied by psychotic symptoms (Lim et al. 1995). Unlike cytomegalovirus and herpes simplex virus, congenital rubella is preventable by vaccination prior to pregnancy.

Cytomegalovirus

Cytomegalovirus is of interest because it is the most common viral infection known to be transmitted in utero and has been associated with delayed neurological effects. The incidence of congenital cytomegalovirus infection is reported to be between 0.2% and 2.2% of all live births (Ho 1991). Among the offspring of pregnancies with serologically documented intrauterine infection, about 5%–10% are

symptomatic at birth, and the majority of these have neuropathological abnormalities and delayed complications, including mental
retardation, delayed psychomotor development, seizures, language delays, and learning disabilities. The period of greatest vulnerability for the fetus is between gestational weeks 4 and 24
(Whitley and Stagno 1991). Like rubella, cytomegalovirus is transmitted from the mother to the fetus via the placenta.

These abnormalities may not manifest until grade school (Raynor 1993). This feature of congenital cytomegalovirus is of relevance to the search for a prenatal viral cause of schizophrenia, since
patients with schizophrenia appear to have had subtle neuropsychiatric developmental disturbances in childhood. However, a series of investigations conducted in the 1970s found no conclusive
evidence of intellectual deficits in individuals with asymptomatic
cytomegalovirus infection (Ho 1991; Kumar et al. 1973; Reynolds et
al. 1974; Saigal et al. 1982).

Herpes Simplex Virus

Herpes simplex virus is a prime example of a viral infection that can
be acquired perinatally; in fact, that is its usual mode of transmission. Transmission occurs when the newborn comes into contact
with infected maternal genital secretions at delivery (Whitley
1990); shedding of the virus is a requisite for transmission. A sexu-
ally transmitted disease, the prevalence of herpes simplex virus is
estimated to be 25%–40% in women of childbearing age; shedding
of the virus occurs in about 0.5%–1.3% of all pregnancies (Whitley
and Stagno 1991). Intrauterine and postnatal infection have also
been described but are much less common. A second important feature of the virus is its predilection for the brain—in particular, for
the temporal lobes, abnormalities of which have been implicated in
schizophrenia. About two-thirds of children with neonatal herpes
simplex virus infection have CNS disease. Unlike rubella and cytomegalovirus, herpes simplex virus infection can be ameliorated
with antiviral treatments, including vidarabine and acyclovir
(Whitley and Stagno 1991).

Pathogenic Mechanisms of Viral Teratogens Affecting CNS Development

Although the specific pathogenic mechanisms responsible for neuro-developmental abnormalities remain unclear (Klein and Remington 1990; Whitley and Stagno 1991), most known viral teratogens disrupt fetal development by direct fetal invasion with or without placental infection (Catalano and Sever 1971; Klein and Remington 1990; Mims 1968). Proposed mechanisms include relatively moderate degrees of cell lysis and tissue necrosis, leading to widespread malformations but less tissue damage than would occur from infection with other viral agents that are less compatible with survival (Klein and Remington 1990; Mims 1968). A second potential pathogenic mechanism for viral teratogens is induction of vasculitis of fetal cerebral arteries, a condition that results in microcephaly, multiple cortical microinfarcts, and foci of calcification (Catalano and Sever 1971). Although rubella produces this inflammatory reaction, it is not yet known whether such vasculitis contributes to the congenital rubella syndrome (Whitley and Stagno 1991).

Viral effects on the placenta might also impair fetal development even if the virus does not invade the fetus (Klein and Remington 1990). Many viruses—including cytomegalovirus, rubella, varicella, and vaccinia—are associated with placental lesions. The mechanism postulated to be responsible for congenital anomalies following placental infection is a generalized vasculitis that compromises placental circulation and leads to hypoxia of fetal organs and tissues (Catalano and Sever 1971).

Contrary to the case for these well-known viral teratogens, direct invasion of the fetus or placenta does not appear to be the pathogenic mechanism for influenza (see subsection below titled "Pathogenic Evidence").

Preliminary Evidence for Prenatal Rubella as a Cause of Schizophrenia

We are currently testing the hypothesis that the risk of schizophrenia is increased after prenatal rubella exposure by following a birth cohort of individuals with congenital rubella. This cohort originally consisted of 243 pregnancies derived from the Rubella Birth Defects Evaluation Project, which was begun after the 1964 rubella epidemic (Chess et al. 1971); these cohort members were followed up through adolescence by Dr. Stella Chess and colleagues. Unlike subjects in prior studies of prenatal viral exposures and schizophrenia, individuals in this birth cohort were serologically documented to have sustained in utero exposure to the virus, either by viral isolation or by IgM-specific antibody in the offspring. We recently discovered that in young adulthood, 70 members of the original birth cohort received a comprehensive diagnostic interview covering lifetime psychiatric disorders, in a study led by Dr. Patricia Cohen. All members of this subsample were of normal intelligence. At present, we are examining the results of these diagnostic assessments and comparing these rubella-exposed subjects with two unexposed cohorts with respect to the occurrence of nonaffective psychosis. Preliminary results suggest an increase in risk of nonaffective psychosis (A. S. Brown, E. S. Susser, P. Cohen, M. Weissman, and S. Greenwald, "Psychosis After Prenatal Exposure to Rubella" [unpublished study], August 1998). To our knowledge, this is the first study to demonstrate a relationship between a serologically documented prenatal exposure and psychosis in adulthood. These findings are of particular interest since rubella, unlike cytomegalovirus and herpes simplex, is preventable by vaccination.

Evidence for and Against Prenatal Influenza as a Cause of CNS Malformations

Of all of the infectious agents examined as putative etiological agents for schizophrenia, influenza exposure during the second trimester of fetal development has emerged as the strongest candidate (Mednick et al. 1988; O'Callaghan et al. 1991). It is therefore of both heuristic and practical value to review evidence of the effects of influenza exposure on CNS development in disorders other than schizophrenia. In contrast to the literature on the infectious agents discussed above, the literature on influenza as a cause of congenital

CNS malformations is controversial. In this section we review epidemiological and pathogenic evidence of CNS effects of influenza on prenatal brain development.

Epidemiological Evidence

A case–control investigation conducted in 1953 by Coffey and Jessop (1955) in Dublin, Ireland, demonstrated a fivefold increased occurrence of congenital malformations in offspring of mothers with "influenza-like" symptoms compared with those without symptoms. In a cohort study conducted during the 1957 Asian influenza epidemic by the same authors, an association was found between prenatal influenza-like illness and neural tube defects (Coffey and Jessop 1959). Two other studies have reported similar findings (Hakosalo and Saxen 1971; Pleydell 1960). More recently, a population-based investigation in Atlanta, Georgia, by Lynberg and colleagues (1994) demonstrated that offspring of mothers reporting flu-like illness accompanied by fever during their pregnancies had a significantly (threefold) increased risk of neural tube defects compared with offspring from pregnancies uncomplicated by flu-like illness. Unlike the previous studies, this investigation included a large sample size, multisource active case ascertainment, and rigorous matching of control subjects to case subjects; it was, however, limited by its use of a broad definition of influenza and the possibility of recall bias.

On the other hand, in large-scale investigations of influenza epidemics between 1957 and 1968 in the United States and in Birmingham, England, Leck and colleagues (Leck 1963, 1971; Leck et al. 1969) found no increased prevalence of CNS malformations following first-trimester influenza exposure. Other studies have similarly failed to find an association between prenatal influenza and CNS malformations (Abramowitz 1958; Campbell 1953; Doll et al. 1960; Elizan et al. 1969; Hardy et al. 1961; Hewitt 1962; Ingalls 1960; Rogers 1972; W. M. Walker and McKee 1959; Wilson and Stein 1969; Wilson et al. 1959).

In summary, the current evidence does not clearly support influenza exposure as a cause of congenital CNS malformations. However, two major limitations could have obscured a potential association in some studies. First, the majority of studies used questionnaires rather than serological data to determine influenza exposure status. In the only study that used serological data to diagnose influenza, about 30% of the total sample had serological evidence of infection but did not receive a clinical diagnosis of influenza (Hardy et al. 1961). Thus, subclinical or mild infections may have been missed in many of the studies. Second, some of the negative studies may have failed to diagnose all cases of congenital neurological malformations, as often occurs in cases of spina bifida occulta, for example, because individuals with spina bifida occulta do not manifest the condition clinically.

Thus, we cannot rule out an effect of prenatal influenza on developmental brain anomalies. The strong association between influenza and cleft lip and other reduction deformities reported in some of the studies reviewed above may be of special significance, given that minor physical anomalies have been repeatedly demonstrated in patients with schizophrenia (Cox and Ludwig 1979; Green et al. 1989) (see Chapter 1, this volume). These abnormalities may reflect a general disruption in fetal development rather than a disruption of CNS development in particular.

Pathogenic Evidence

Preclinical studies have demonstrated that prenatal influenza infection can cause congenital malformations. Relative to the case for the viruses discussed above, however, less is known regarding whether influenza infection acts directly or indirectly in producing these malformations. Inoculation of chick embryos with influenza virus at 24 hours of incubation has been demonstrated (K. P. Johnson et al. 1971; R. T. Johnson 1972) to result in micrencephaly and neural tube anomalies, including abnormalities of flexure and failure of closure (myeloschisis). These anomalies were not associated with necrosis, and mitotic activity appeared normal (R. T. Johnson 1972). In addition, there was no evidence of influenza virus in neural ectoderm or surrounding mesenchymal cells; rather, viral antigen was found in chorionic and amnionic membranes and nonneural ectoderm as well as in the primitive myocardium and gut (K. P. Johnson et al. 1971). The authors suggested that the viral infection may have altered the relationship between extraneural tissues and the neural tube (K. P. Johnson et al. 1971). Studies of pregnant mice inoculated with influenza virus immediately after mating demonstrated cephalic abnormalities, growth retardation, and fetal resorption in the offspring (Adams et al. 1956; Heath et al. 1956). Influenza virus was recovered only from fetuses infected late in gestation and removed prior to delivery, a finding suggesting that the placental barrier likely prevents infection during early pregnancy (Siem et al. 1960).

While rubella and herpes simplex virus have been demonstrated to directly invade the placenta and fetus, there is little evidence that this route of infection occurs with influenza virus. Evidence in humans for direct fetal infection by the influenza virus is scant, with only a small number of case reports documenting isolation of the virus in placental or fetal tissue from infected mothers (Kilbourne 1987; Yawn et al. 1971). The immunological data are also equivocal. In one study, the cord sera from eight infants of mothers with documented maternal influenza during the second and third trimesters had no evidence of elevated immunoglobulin M (IgM) levels to influenza antigen (Monif et al. 1972). However, another study demonstrated responses to influenza A viral antigens in cord blood lymphocytes of infants from exposed pregnancies, suggesting that fetal infection occurred prior to delivery (Ruben and Thompson 1981).

Potential Causal Pathways of Prenatal Influenza in Schizophrenia

Whereas the pathogenesis of most known viral teratogens appears to involve direct infection, it appears that if prenatal influenza is a causal agent in schizophrenia, its effects are not direct, but instead involve a variety of mediating factors. One must also consider potential coincident factors that interact with influenza. We highlight this issue next, as it represents a critical area for future research.

Mediation of Effect

One possible mediating factor is the use of over-the-counter or pre-scribed flu remedies, which are commonly taken during preg-nancy. If these medications have teratogenic potential, adverse fetal outcomes could arise. In the large Atlanta, Georgia, study by Lynberg and colleagues (1994) reported earlier in this chapter, a fourfold increase in risk of spina bifida and of total neural tube de-fects was found among offspring of women who medicated their influenza and fever compared with those who did not report epi-sodes of influenza or fever. However, there was no increase in risk of total neural tube defects in those with influenza who took no medications compared with those without influenza or fever. Of note, aspirin was associated with a sixfold increase in total neural tube defects, and decongestants with an eightfold increase. How-ever, because women with more severe influenza symptoms are also those most likely to take medication, these findings could have resulted from a relationship between illness severity and neural tube defects. In addition, sample sizes of individuals in each medi-cation group were small, and the comparison group consisted of pregnant women without flu or fever, thus confounding the effects of medication and influenza on risk of total neural tube defects. Nonetheless, if medication-taking behavior and specific flu reme-dies differed between countries, a teratogenic effect of flu remedies might explain conflicting findings from epidemiological studies at-tempting to link influenza epidemics with schizophrenia in ex-posed offspring (Erlenmeyer-Kimling et al. 1994; Mednick et al. 1988; O'Callaghan et al. 1991; Susser et al. 1994).

A second potential mediating factor is hyperthermia. Several preclinical and epidemiological investigations have implicated hyperthermia as a cause of CNS anomalies, including neural tube defects. Pregnant rats and guinea pigs exposed to hot environ-ments have an increased risk of bearing offspring with nervous sys-tem defects (Edwards 1968, 1969), and maternal hyperthermia is associated with CNS defects in chicks and mice (Adams et al. 1956; Heath et al. 1956). Hyperthermia also disrupts neural-groove clo-sure (Kilham and Ferm 1976; Skreb and Frank 1963). Epidemiological studies of pregnant women have linked use of saunas, hot tubs, electric blankets, and fever due to infection with an increased rate of neural tube defects among the offspring (Adams et al. 1956; Layde et al. 1980; Milunsky et al. 1992; Shiota 1982).

However, Lynberg and colleagues (1994) demonstrated a significantly increased risk of neural tube defects among pregnancies complicated by at least 2 days of influenza, irrespective of whether the illness was complicated by fever. In this study, fever from other causes was not associated with a higher rate of neural tube defects. Notwithstanding, the number of pregnancies in which fever from other causes occurred was small, and the severity and duration of fever secondary to influenza could have been higher than fever secondary to other infections.

Other potential mediating factors include metabolic derangements, circulating toxins, anoxia, and an abnormal maternal immune response (see Chapter 4, this volume).

Modification of Effect

Two factors that might accompany maternal influenza and that could interact to increase risk of schizophrenia are nutritional deprivation and a concurrent infection. Poor maternal nutrition might occur either independently of the infection or secondary to the infectious process. In studies of the Dutch Hunger Winter, prenatal exposure to severe famine was associated with a twofold increase in the risk of schizophrenia in exposed offspring (Susser and Lin 1992; Susser et al. 1996). Since anorexia is a common symptom of influenza, pregnant women are likely to restrict their intake of food during the infection. If this nutritional deficit coincides with a critical period of fetal development, it might interact with the influenza episode to increase the risk of schizophrenia.

Moreover, influenza is not uncommonly associated with secondary infections, often bacterial, as a result of compromised resistance. Often, such secondary infections are more severe than the primary infections. Thus, an influenza epidemic may be merely a marker of a secondary epidemic by a co-infecting organism. Alternatively, influenza and the co-infecting organism may interact in increasing the risk for schizophrenia.

Strategies for Future Research

It is critical to develop research strategies to address and resolve conflicting findings regarding prenatal influenza and schizophrenia and to ascertain suspected mediating and interacting factors. Several potentially useful strategies are discussed below.

Epidemiological Studies

Previous studies of prenatal influenza exposure and schizophrenia have yielded conflicting findings. One potential explanation for these discrepancies relates to inadequate ascertainment of both exposure and outcome, which would tend to underestimate the size of a potential association. These studies defined as "exposed" those cohorts that were in utero during an influenza epidemic rather than using more precise individual measures, and used diagnoses from hospital registries rather than those based on chart reviews and direct interviews.

Our group is actively pursuing two research studies that will address these limitations: the Prenatal Determinants of Schizophrenia (PDS) study and the Congenital Rubella in Schizophrenia (CRIS) study.

Prenatal Determinants of Schizophrenia Study

The PDS study is a birth cohort study of nearly 20,000 pregnancies of women enrolled in the Child Health and Development Study in Oakland, California between 1959 and 1966. The offspring of these women are currently being followed up via direct interviews to diagnose schizophrenia cases. The advantages of the PDS study include the use of exposure data from individuals rather than groups, precise documentation of exposure, and comprehensive and rigorous diagnostic assessment of potential schizophrenia cases from a representative cohort. A unique strength of the study is the presence of stored serum samples from pregnant mothers throughout gestation, which will permit assessment of influenza exposure using serial antibody titers.

Congenital Rubella Schizophrenia Study

We are currently extending our efforts to examine the relation of other prenatal viruses to schizophrenia. One such virus, described earlier, is rubella. In the CRIS study, a follow-up study of the Rubella Birth Defects Evaluation Project, we are conducting more extensive diagnostic interviews and brain imaging on cohort members and family history assessments for psychotic disorders in the relatives of the cohort members. This study will enable us to examine genetic–viral interactions in the etiology of schizophrenia and to explore structural and functional brain abnormalities in relation to prenatal rubella exposure. Furthermore, this comprehensive data set will permit exploration of potential mediating and interacting factors, including medication use, nutritional intake, and co-infecting organisms.

Preclinical Studies

Further support for plausibility could derive from animal studies examining whether gestational influenza induces neuropathology similar to that found in schizophrenia. Such an animal model could also be used to examine the pathogenesis of infection, including direct versus indirect mechanisms, and the effects of the timing of infection on the developing brain.

The design of such a study would be relatively straightforward. Samples of pregnant rats would be inoculated with influenza virus at various stages of gestation. The offspring would be sacrificed and the brains examined for evidence of influenza virus and for structural anomalies, both gross (i.e., ventriculomegaly, diminished hippocampal volume) and ultrastructural (i.e., cellular disarray, migration disturbances). Another series of experiments could specifically examine the contribution of immune-mediated alterations to structural brain anomalies. In this design, pregnant rats would receive an influenza vaccine to stimulate the production of antibody without inducing high fever or exposing the mother or fetus to live virus. Mother and fetus could also be assessed for influenza autoantibody.

Conclusion

Evidence from neuropathological and epidemiological studies supports the plausibility of prenatal viral infection as a risk factor for schizophrenia. Individuals with congenital viral syndromes and schizophrenia are concordant with respect to several pathological features indicative of early developmental insults. Rubella, cytomegalovirus, and herpes simplex virus may serve as useful models to illustrate specific effects of prenatal viral infection, which may have implications for understanding gestational viral exposures in the etiopathogenesis of schizophrenia. Prenatal influenza, the strongest potential viral candidate for schizophrenia, may be a cause of developmental brain anomalies, although the literature on this subject is conflicting. If prenatal influenza plays a role in the etiology of schizophrenia, its effects likely result from mediating or interacting factors rather than from direct fetal invasion of the virus. Future epidemiological research may resolve conflicting findings on prenatal influenza in schizophrenia, and further preclinical work may lead to an animal model of gestational effects of influenza on brain development.

The identification of a prenatal viral agent responsible for even a small proportion of schizophrenia cases would profoundly affect our understanding of the pathogenesis of the illness, even among cases resulting from other factors. Equally important would be the potential ramifications of this new knowledge on the primary prevention of schizophrenia, which might one day include a rigorous program of vaccinations in women prior to pregnancy and other public health measures. Although much work remains to be done, the search for prenatal viruses as causative agents in schizophrenia is an endeavor that holds great promise for the field and offers hope for victims of this devastating illness.

References

Abramowitz LJ: The effect of Asian influenza on pregnancy. S Afr Med J 32:1155–1156, 1958

Achs R, Harper RG, Siegel M: Unusual dermatoglyphic findings associated with rubella embryopathy. N Engl J Med 274:148–150, 1966

Adams JM, Heath HD, Imagawa DT, et al: Viral infections in the embryo. Am J Dis Child 92:109–114, 1956

Barr CE, Mednick SA, Munk-Jorgensen P: Exposure to influenza epidemics during gestation and adult schizophrenia: a 40-year study. Arch Gen Psychiatry 47:869–874, 1990

Campbell WAB: Influenza in early pregnancy: effects on the foetus. Lancet 1:173–174, 1953

Catalano LW Jr, Sever JL: The role of viruses as causes of congenital defects. Annu Rev Microbiol 25:255–282, 1971

Chess S, Korn SJ, Fernandez PB: Psychiatric Disorders of Children With Congenital Rubella. New York, Brunner/Mazel, 1971

Coffey VP, Jessop WJE: Congenital abnormalities—6th series. Ir J Med Sci 349:30–46, 1955

Coffey VP, Jessop WJE: Maternal influenza and congenital deformities: a prospective study. Lancet 2:935–938, 1959

Cox SM, Ludwig AM: Neurological soft signs and psychopathology, I: findings in schizophrenia. J Nerv Ment Dis 167:161–165, 1979

Desmond MM, Wilson GS, Melnick JL, et al: Congenital rubella encephalitis: course and early sequelae. J Pediatr 71:311–331, 1967

Desmond MM, Montgomery JR, Melnick JL, et al: Congenital rubella encephalitis: effect on growth and early development. Am J Dis Child 118:30–31, 1969

Doll R, Hill AB, Sakula J: Asian influenza in pregnancy and congenital defects. British Journal of Preventive and Social Medicine 14:167–172, 1960

Edwards MJ: Congenital malformations in the rat following induced hyperthermia during gestation. Teratology 1:173–175, 1968

Edwards MJ: Congenital defects in guinea-pigs: prenatal retardation of brain growth of guinea-pigs following hyperthermia during gestation. Teratology 2:329–336, 1969

Elizan TS, Ajero-Froehlich L, Fabiyi A, et al: Viral infection in pregnancy and congenital CNS malformations in man. Arch Neurol 20:115–119, 1969

Erlenmeyer-Kimling L, Folnegovic Z, Hrabak-Zerjavic Boracic B, et al: Schizophrenia and prenatal exposure to the 1957 A2 influenza epidemic in Croatia. Am J Psychiatry 151:1496–1498, 1994

Fish B, Marcus J, Hans SL, et al: Infants at risk for schizophrenia: sequelae of a genetic neurointegrative defect. Arch Gen Psychiatry 49:221–235, 1992

Green MF, Satz P, Gruen DJ, et al: Minor physical anomalies in schizophrenia. Schizophr Bull 15:91–99, 1989

Gregg NM: Congenital cataract following German measles in the mother. Transactions of the Ophthalmological Society of Australia (BMA) 3: 35–46, 1942

Gregg NM, Beavis WR, Heseltine M, et al: The occurrence of congenital defects in children following maternal rubella during pregnancy. Med J Aust 2:122–126, 1945

Hakosalo JK, Saxen L: Influenza epidemic and congenital defects. Lancet 2:1346–1347, 1971

Hardy JMB, Azarowicz EN, Mannini A, et al: The effect of Asian influenza on the outcome of pregnancy, Baltimore, 1957–58. Am J Public Health 51:1182–1188, 1961

Heath HD, Shear HH, Imagawa DT, et al: Teratogenic effects of herpes simplex, vaccinia, influenza A (NWS), and distemper virus infections on early chick embryos. Proc Soc Exp Biol Med 92:675–682, 1956

Hewitt D: A study of temporal variations in the risk of fetal malformation and death. Am J Public Health 52:1676–1688, 1962

Ho M: Cytomegalovirus: Biology and Infection. New York, Plenum, 1991

Ingalls TH: Prenatal human ecology. Am J Public Health 50:50–54, 1960

Johnson KP, Klasnja R, Johnson RT: Neural tube defects of chick embryos: an indirect result of influenza A virus infection. J Neuropathol Exp Neurol 30:68–74, 1971

Johnson RT: Effects of viral infection on the developing nervous system. N Engl J Med 287:599–604, 1972

Jones P, Rodgers B, Murray R, et al: Child developmental risk factors for adult schizophrenia in the British 1946 birth cohort. Lancet 344:1398–1402, 1994

Kilbourne ED: Influenza. New York, Plenum, 1987

Kilham L, Ferm VH: Exencephaly in fetal hamsters following exposure to hyperthermia. Teratology 14:323–336, 1976

Klein JO, Remington JS: Current concepts of infections of the fetus and newborn infant, in Infectious Diseases of the Fetus and Newborn Infant, 3rd Edition. Edited by Remington JS, Klein JO. Philadelphia, PA, WB Saunders, 1990, pp 1–16

Kumar ML, Nankervis GA, Gold E: Inapparent congenital cytomegalovirus infections: a follow-up study. N Engl J Med 288:1370–1372, 1973

Kunugi H, Nanko S, Takei N, et al: Schizophrenia following in utero exposure to the 1957 influenza epidemics in Japan. Am J Psychiatry 152: 450–452, 1995

Layde PM, Edmonds LD, Erickson JD: Maternal fever and neural tube defects. Teratology 21:105–108, 1980

Leck I: Incidence of malformation following influenza epidemics. British Journal of Preventive and Social Medicine 17:70–80, 1963

Leck I: Further tests of the hypothesis that influenza in pregnancy causes malformations. Health Services Mental Health Administration Health Reports 86:265–269, 1971

Leck I, Hay S, Witte JJ, et al: Malformations recorded on birth certificates following A2 influenza epidemics. Public Health Rep 84:971–979, 1969

Lim KO, Beal M, Harvey RL, et al: Brain dysmorphology in adults with congenital rubella plus schizophrenialike symptoms. Biol Psychiatry 37:764–776, 1995

Lynberg MC, Khoury MJ, Lu X, et al: Maternal flu, fever, and the risk of neural tube defects: a population-based case-control study. Am J Epidemiol 140:244–255, 1994

Mednick SA, Machon RA, Huttunen MO, et al: Adult schizophrenia following prenatal exposure to an influenza epidemic. Arch Gen Psychiatry 45:189–192, 1988

Milunsky A, Ulcickas M, Rothman KJ, et al: Maternal heat exposure and neural tube defects. JAMA 268:882–885, 1992

Mims CA: Pathogenesis of viral infections of the fetus. Prog Med Virol 10:194–237, 1968

Monif GRG, Sowards DL, Eitzman DV: Serologic and immunologic evaluation of neonates following maternal influenza infection during the second and third trimesters of gestation. Am J Obstet Gynecol 114: 239–242, 1972

O'Callaghan E, Sham PC, Takei N, et al: Schizophrenia after prenatal exposure to 1957 A2 influenza epidemic. Lancet 337:1248–1250, 1991

O'Callaghan E, Sham PC, Takei N, et al: The relationship of schizophrenic births to 16 infectious diseases. Br J Psychiatry 165:353–356, 1994

Pleydell MD: Anencephaly and other congenital abnormalities: an epidemiological study in Northamptonshire. BMJ 1:309–315, 1960

Purvis-Smith SG, Menser MA: Genetic and environmental influences on digital dermatoglyphics in congenital rubella. Pediatr Res 7:215–219, 1973

Purvis-Smith SG, Hayes K, Menser MA: Dermatoglyphics in children with prenatal cytomegalovirus infection. Lancet 2:976–977, 1972

Raynor BD: Cytomegalovirus infection in pregnancy. Semin Perinatol 17: 394–402, 1993

Reynolds DW, Stagno S, Stubbs G, et al: Inapparent congenital cytomegalovirus infection with elevated cord IgM levels. N Engl J Med 290:291–296, 1974

Rogers SC: Influenza and congenital abnormalities. Lancet 1:261, 1972

Ruben FL, Thompson DS: Cord blood lymphocyte in vitro responses to influenza A antigens after an epidemic of influenza A/Port Chalmers/73 {H3N2}. Am J Obstet Gynecol 141:443–446, 1981

Saigal S, Lunyk O, Larke RPB, et al: The outcome in children with congenital cytomegalovirus infection. Am J Dis Child 136:896–901, 1982

Sham PC, O'Callaghan E, Takei N, et al: Schizophrenia following prenatal exposure to influenza epidemics between 1939 and 1960. Br J Psychiatry 160:461–466, 1992

Shiota K: Neural tube defects and maternal hyperthermia in early pregnancy: epidemiology in a human embryo population. Am J Med Genet 12:281–288, 1982

Siem RA, Ly H, Imagawa DT, et al: Influenza virus infections in pregnant mice. J Neuropathol Exp Neurol 19:125–129, 1960

Skreb N, Frank Z: Developmental abnormalities in the rat induced by heat shock. Journal of Embryology and Experimental Morphology 11: 445–447, 1963

Susser ES, Lin SP: Schizophrenia after prenatal exposure to the Dutch Hunger Winter of 1944–45. Arch Gen Psychiatry 49:983–988, 1992

Susser E, Lin SP, Brown AS, et al: No relation between risk of schizophrenia and prenatal exposure to influenza in Holland. Am J Psychiatry 151:922–924, 1994

Susser ES, Neugebauer R, Hoek HW, et al: Schizophrenia after prenatal famine: further evidence. Arch Gen Psychiatry 53:25–31, 1996

Torrey EF, Rawlings R, Waldman IN: Schizophrenic births and viral diseases in two states. Schizophr Res 1:73–77, 1988

Waddington JL: Schizophrenia: developmental neuroscience and pathobiology. Lancet 341:531–536, 1993

Walker EF, Savoie T, Davis D: Neuromotor precursors of schizophrenia. Schizophr Bull 20:441–451, 1994

Walker WM, McKee AP: Asian influenza in pregnancy: relationship to fetal anomalies. Obstet Gynecol 13:394–398, 1959

Watson CG, Kucala T, Tilleskjor C, et al: Schizophrenic birth seasonality in relation to the incidence of infectious diseases and temperature extremes. Arch Gen Psychiatry 41:85–90, 1984

Whitley RJ: Herpes simplex virus infections, in Infectious Diseases of the Fetus and Newborn Infant, 3rd Edition. Edited by Remington JS, Klein JO. Philadelphia, PA, WB Saunders, 1990, pp 282–305

Whitley RJ, Stagno S: Perinatal viral infections, in Infections of the Central Nervous System. Edited by Scheld WM, Whitley RJ, Durack DT. New York, Raven, 1991, pp 167–200

Wilson MG, Stein AM: Teratogenic effects of Asian influenza. JAMA 210:336–337, 1969

Wilson MG, Heins HL, Imagawa DT, et al: Teratogenic effects of Asian influenza. JAMA 171:638–641, 1959

Yawn DH, Pyeatte JC, Joseph JM, et al: Transplacental transfer of influenza virus. JAMA 1216:1022–1023, 1971

Part III

Prenatal Nutritional Exposures

Chapter 6

The Dutch Famine Studies: Prenatal Nutritional Deficiency and Schizophrenia

Hans W. Hoek, M.D., Ph.D., Alan S. Brown, M.D., and
Ezra S. Susser, M.D., Dr.P.H.

G iven that prenatal nutritional deficiencies are among the most common causes of neurodevelopmental disorders (Brown et al. 1996), prenatal nutrition represents a logical starting point in the search for causes of neurodevelopmental schizophrenia. Indeed, a relationship between prenatal nutritional deficiency and the risk of schizophrenia in offspring was proposed as early as the 1950s (Pasamanick et al. 1956). Until recently, however, the nutritional hypothesis was not tested. The difficulties of obtaining data on exposure to prenatal nutritional deficiency on the one hand, and data on psychiatric outcomes many years later in adulthood on the other, proved insurmountable.

This chapter describes the Dutch famine studies, which provided the first test of the nutritional hypothesis. In the Dutch Hunger Winter at the end of World War II, a combination of circumstances, some of them tragic, created the conditions of a natural experiment. Unlike other famines, the Dutch famine struck at a precisely circumscribed time and place and in a society able to document the timing and severity of the nutritional deprivation as well

This work was supported in part by the Theodore and Vada Stanley Foundation. Support was also provided by The Hague Psychiatric Institute and Leiden University, The Netherlands (H. W. Hoek) and the New York State Psychiatric Institute/Columbia University, U.S.A. (E. Susser, A. Brown).

as the effects on fertility and health. As a result, it was possible to define sequential birth cohorts exposed to famine at specific times in gestation as well as to define birth cohorts who were not exposed to prenatal famine but who in other ways were highly similar to the exposed cohorts. Moreover, because the Dutch maintained comprehensive military and health records over a long period after the famine, it was possible to compare the incidence of neurodevelopmental disorders in adulthood in the exposed and unexposed cohorts.

The investigation of neurodevelopmental disorders in the Dutch famine cohorts actually represents not a single study but three "generations" of studies (Susser et al. 1998a). Taken together, these have provided, and are continuing to uncover, a wealth of information on the neuropsychiatric outcomes resulting from deficits in prenatal nutrition. The investigations were initiated in the original Dutch Famine Study by Stein and colleagues (1975), who aimed primarily to relate prenatal famine to adult mental competence. A "second generation" of studies extended this work to relate prenatal famine to schizophrenia-spectrum disorders (Hoek et al. 1996, 1998; Susser and Lin 1992; Susser et al. 1996). In a "third generation" of studies, still in progress, we are examining the interrelationship between prenatal famine and genetic vulnerability in the origins of schizophrenia (Hoek et al. 1994, 1998).

In this chapter we first review the historical circumstances of the Dutch Hunger Winter that created this unique natural experiment. The following sections review, in turn, the original Dutch Famine Study on which the later work on schizophrenia was based, the second-generation schizophrenia studies, and the ongoing work of the third generation of research.

The Dutch Hunger Winter of 1944–1945

The Netherlands, a small country, is customarily divided by the points of a compass into four regions. The West is the commercial and industrial heart of the country. The North is the "breadbasket" of the country and is separated from the West by the Ijsselmeer.

South of the great rivers of the Rhine estuary lies another agricultural region. Finally, the East is a mixed region of somewhat less economic importance.

In 1945, the population density of The Netherlands was the highest in the world and was twice as high in the industrial western part of the country as in the other regions. Although the western region had only one-fifth of the total land area, half the people in the country (approximately 5 million) lived there. Five of the cities in the western region—namely, Amsterdam, Rotterdam, The Hague, Utrecht, and Haarlem—were the largest in The Netherlands.

The Netherlands Before the Famine

Because of its high population density, The Netherlands depended on imports to maintain its food supply. Heavy imports of grain, oilseed, and cattlefeed went to the dairy farms, and these in turn produced milk, butter, cheese, meat, and eggs, much of which was exported (Breunis 1946; Dols and van Arcken 1946).

Standards of public health were high before World War II. The overall mortality rate of 8.7 per 1,000 in 1939 was low, and the infant mortality and tuberculosis mortality rates were among the lowest in the world (Banning 1946). Food was plentiful, as indicated by the consumption of calories and protein (Dols and van Arcken 1946). Social and health services were widely available. Community care for mental disorders, a movement pioneered in The Netherlands, had its beginnings before World War II.

The outbreak of World War II found the Dutch prepared to safeguard their food supplies. Plans had been made to adjust agricultural production for each contingency and to introduce a system of rationing. Immediately on the outbreak of war in September 1939, imports of animal feed stopped and the rationing of animal feed was begun. In May 1940, The Netherlands was occupied by the Germans and the rationing of foods for the Dutch people began. By April 1941, virtually all foods were being rationed. Up to the end of 1943, the rationing successfully ensured basic nutrition for the population, with a well-balanced average daily ration in the range of 6,380–8,400 kilojoules (kJ) (1,500–2,000 kilocalories [kcal]).

During 1944, however, conditions deteriorated. Increasingly, the food that was produced in The Netherlands was being diverted to meet the food needs of the occupation forces and the German population (Bourne 1943; Burger et al. 1948; Dols and van Arcken 1946). Thus, the food supplies were already marginal before the onset of the Dutch Hunger Winter in October of 1944.

The Hunger Winter

The final episode of the war in The Netherlands began in September 1944. The Allied forces entered the country, but two large branches of the Rhine barred their advance on the main industrial centers of Germany. In a daring operation that included a paratroop drop behind the German lines, the Allies attempted to seize the strategic bridges that spanned the river at Nijmegen and Arnhem.

The Allied paratroop drop ended in disaster in the forests of Arnhem. As the fighting continued, both Arnhem and Nijmegen were severely battered and the people evacuated. By mid-November, the Allied forces had liberated The Netherlands south of the Rhine, but they had failed to take the crucial bridges. Most of The Netherlands, including the industrial West, remained under German occupation. Major fighting in that sector of the front ceased until the end of March 1945.

During the battle, the Dutch government in exile in London had broadcast an appeal for a general railroad strike to impede the German defenses. Despite threats of reprisal, the Dutch rail workers had brought rail traffic to a standstill. In retaliation, the German occupation forces then imposed the reprisal they had threatened, an embargo on all transport, including food supplies.

The food situation in the cities of the West, already difficult in September when the Allied drive on the Rhine began, worsened with the embargo on transport imposed by the German occupation force. As the food shortage became acute, the Occupation Authority relented a little and lifted the total embargo to permit the use of water transport to bring food from the agricultural North to the cities of the West. But winter was both unusually early and severe in 1944–1945. Before much could be done, the canals had frozen and the barges could not move.

While the war continued, other circumstances exacerbated the shortage of food in the West. The means of transport were increasingly commandeered by the Occupation Authority. Many farmers were drafted. Large tracts of the country were inundated by the breaking of the sea dikes to delay an Allied invasion, and much farmland was given up to the construction of airfields and fortifications. In all, 230,000 hectares were rendered useless for agriculture. Gradually the food shortage in the West evolved into a severe famine.

Regional Distribution of the Famine

The famine was restricted to the half of the population residing in the West. The shortages in the other parts of the country were of much briefer duration and did not amount to persisting famine with starvation. In the West, the famine was largely a phenomenon of the cities and towns (Figure 6–1). Rural people produced food for their own subsistence, even at the height of the famine.

The regional differences can be illustrated by the prices of food on the black market during the famine (De Jong 1981). In October 1944 in The Hague, the black market price for a kilo of flour was 7 Dutch florin (as compared with the official price of 0.25 florin); by April 1945, that price had risen to 50 florin. By comparison, in the largest city in the North, Groningen, the April 1945 black market price for the same kilo of flour was still less than 1 florin.

Increasing Intensity of the Famine

The famine progressively intensified in the West, or famine region, with rations declining to extremely low levels between February and May 1945. In the last months of the Hunger Winter, the average daily intake of the official ration was below 4,200 kJ (1,000 kcal), and bread, potatoes, and sugar beets formed almost the entire ration (see Figure 6–2). Rations were commonly supplemented by

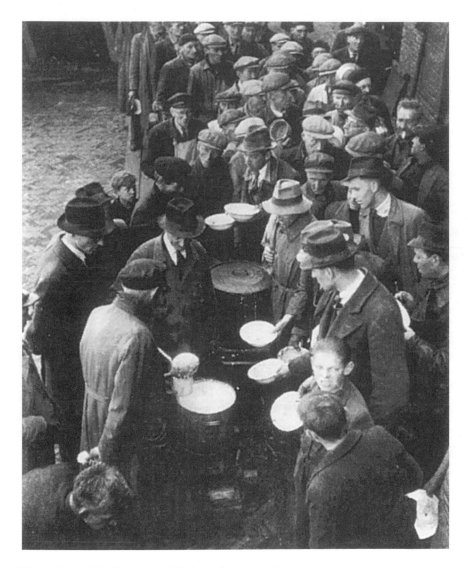

Figure 6–1.   Food was provided via the eating-houses.
Source.   National Institute for War Documentation, Amsterdam.

unusual foods such as tulip bulbs (Figure 6–3). The famine reached its peak during the 4 weeks before the actual liberation on May 7, 1945, when the advance of the Allied forces had completely separated the West from the rest of the country (De Jong 1981; Slager et al. 1985; Stein et al. 1975). The famine conditions continued until

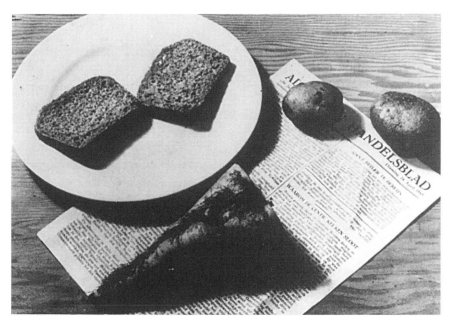

Figure 6–2. The average daily food ration.
Source. National Institute for War Documentation, Amsterdam.

several days after the official liberation day of The Netherlands, May 5, 1945 (De Jong 1981; Slager et al. 1985).

Effects on Fertility

The famine had dramatic and well-documented effects on fertility (Stein et al. 1975). In The Hague's municipal hospital, 60% of the female employees had disturbances in their menstrual periods during the famine (De Jong 1981). Many men became impotent; there were hardly any sexual crimes during the famine (De Jong 1981). The lowered fertility of the population during the worst of the famine was reflected in a nadir in the birth rate in the West of The Netherlands 9 months after the famine; the birth rate fell to less than 50% of previous levels. The decline in fertility was less in the upper than in the lower classes; this was no doubt due to the fact that the upper classes had more access to nonration food from sources such as the black market.

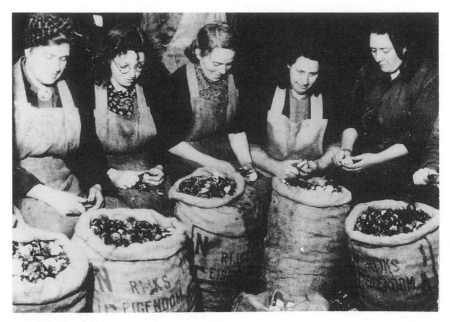

Figure 6–3. In January the eating-houses also started to process beets and bulbs for dietary consumption. The Council of Nutrition furnished recipes to help make these items more palatable.
Source.   National Institute for War Documentation, Amsterdam.

Mortality and Morbidity

Of the 3.5 million inhabitants of the western part of The Netherlands, at least 22,000 people (De Jong 1981) died because of the famine (Figure 6–4). The exact number of hunger-edema patients is unknown, but these patients filled the hospitals. When the famine ended in May 1945, approximately 200,000 people were estimated to be ill from starvation.

The Original Dutch Famine Study

The original Dutch Famine Study of Stein and colleagues (1975) was designed to trace, in mature individuals, the neurodevelopmental effects of prenatal exposure to famine. The neurodevelopmental outcome of central interest was mild mental retardation or depressed IQ. A strong association between social conditions and

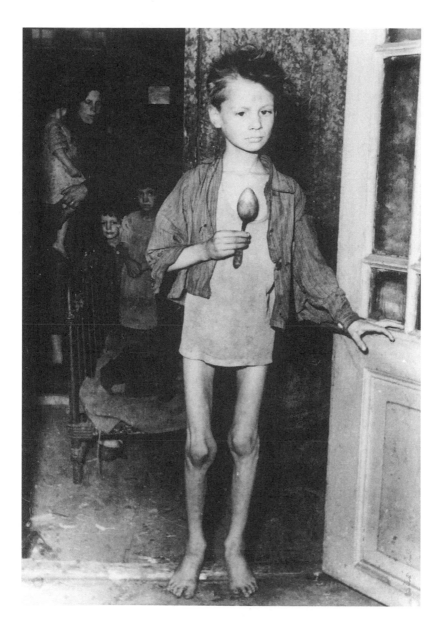

Figure 6–4. In exchange for a few children's shirts and some bread, the photographer Martinus Meijboom received permission to take some pictures of the Holvast family with their many children, living in Amsterdam. This is "Henkie," the oldest child. The two youngest children did not survive the Hunger Winter, although Henkie did.
Source. National Institute for War Documentation, Amsterdam.

the mental performance of mature adults had already been documented. The broad question posed by this study was how much of that association could be explained by the variation across society of prenatal nutrition. The more specific question tested was whether severe but balanced deficiency in the nutrients supplied to groups of mothers during any stage of pregnancy had detectable effects on the mental abilities of the offspring when they reached maturity.

The strategy the authors adopted to answer this question anticipated the strategy of the later schizophrenia study, and, in addition, their findings provided the rationale for that study. Therefore, we describe here the design and the findings of the original study.

Design

To examine the effects of prenatal famine on mental performance, the authors used a cohort design. Such a design begins with a study group of individuals who have experienced the hypothetical causal factor; the proportion who develop the manifestation of interest is then identified. A control group of persons who have not experienced the causal factor is selected for comparison; among them, too, the proportion who develop the manifestation is identified. A significant excess of the manifestation in the study group compared with the control group supports the hypothesis.

Exposed and Unexposed Cohorts

About 40,000 individuals were exposed to the Hunger Winter at some point in gestation. The clear demarcation of the famine in time and place provided a key to identifying exposed individuals. Any individual could be classified in the group exposed to famine during a specific period in gestation if he or she was born within a given calendar period in the famine-stricken areas. This calendar period could be determined from the known duration of the famine and the normal duration of pregnancy. By the same token, all those born outside these limits of time and place could be classified as unexposed.

Neurodevelopmental Outcomes

A follow-up of all exposed and unexposed individuals in these cohorts was bound to prove laborious and, quite likely, impractical. Therefore, the authors searched among institutions of The Netherlands for completed and stored data sets that could serve as epidemiological checkpoints in the life cycles of all of the affected individuals. The data had to meet two fundamental criteria: 1) the members of the cohorts at risk who passed through the checkpoint must have been systematically rated in terms of mental performance, and 2) date and place of birth must have been recorded for each individual, as required to assign individuals to exposed and unexposed groups.

By far the best checkpoint proved to be military induction data on males at age 18 years. In the Dutch military draft system at the time of the study, the names of all men, when they reached the age of 18 years, were sent forward from the population registers kept by each community to the military authorities. With the exception of a few statutory exemptions, amounting to about 3% of individuals in each age group, every man was called up for a thorough and standardized medical and psychological examination. Although men institutionalized for mental disorders or other disabilities were not required to appear in person, they, too, were entered into the military record. Each institution with a resident population was required to notify the Dutch military authorities about the health and mental status of male inmates of requisite age and to provide documented support for the clinical opinions and diagnoses proffered.

The investigators obtained the cooperation of the Dutch military authorities for the use of the military induction data. The military made available the complete results of the induction medical examinations, already coded and transferred to computer tapes, for all Dutch men born in the years 1944 through 1946. These data included detailed measures of mental performance as well as International Classification of Diseases (ICD) diagnoses of all health disorders among the inductees.

Findings

There were two key findings among the military inductees in this original study, each of which was somewhat surprising at the time. First, there were no detectable effects of prenatal famine on IQ or on numerous other measures of mental performance. The authors concluded that acute prenatal nutritional deprivation cannot be considered a factor in the social distribution of mental competence among surviving adults in well-nourished industrial societies. Chronic nutritional deficiency may yet play a role, however; poor maternal, prenatal, and postnatal nutrition often occur in poorly nourished populations.

Second, the single health disorder that varied in frequency with prenatal exposure to famine was congenital anomalies of the central nervous system (CNS). The excess of CNS anomalies was detectable only among birth cohorts conceived during the peak months of the famine, approximately February–April 1945; thus, it was an effect of exposure in early gestation and was evident only in the most severely exposed birth cohorts.

The latter finding provided the rationale for the second generation of research on schizophrenia after prenatal exposure to famine. The birth cohorts with an excess of CNS anomalies were known to have suffered disturbances in brain development as a result of a prenatal exposure. Therefore, a study of schizophrenia in these cohorts represented a logical step in the search for etiologies of neurodevelopmental schizophrenia.

Studies of Schizophrenia and Related Disorders

The schizophrenia studies in the Dutch famine cohorts were initiated with an explicit and specific hypothesis in mind. Motivated by the findings of the original study described above, we aimed to test whether early prenatal exposure to famine was associated not only with various congenital CNS anomalies but also with an increased risk of schizophrenia (Susser and Lin 1992; Susser et al. 1996, 1998a). Thus, our a priori hypothesis was that an increased risk of schizophrenia would be found among the birth cohorts conceived at the height of the famine and exhibiting an excess of congenital neural defects.

The overall design of the second-generation studies conformed closely with the design of the original study. Further precision was achieved, however, in the definition of the exposed birth cohorts. In the original study, the authors explored the effects of exposure at all periods of gestation and defined birth cohorts as exposed to prenatal famine in early gestation, midgestation, or late gestation based on the documented food rations and famine severity. By contrast, the second-generation studies focused specifically on the birth cohorts that had shown an excess of CNS anomalies after exposure in early gestation and aimed to define the early gestational exposure as precisely as possible.

Schizophrenia

In the schizophrenia study, three criteria were used to define the exposed birth cohort in the cities of the West that were affected by the famine. The first criterion was low food rations during the first trimester of gestation. The birth cohorts of August–December 1945 met this criterion. The second criterion was conception at the height of the famine, as indicated by adverse health effects in the general population. The later-born individuals among the birth cohorts of August–December 1945 (born October 15–December 31) met this criterion, but the earlier-born ones (August 1–October 14) did not. The third criterion was a detectable excess of congenital neural defects. To apply this criterion, we returned to the data of the original study and reanalyzed the findings. The birth cohorts of 1944–1946 were divided into 2-month periods. However, the period of May–December 1945 was divided into May–July, August 1–October 14, and October 15–December 31. For each of the 17 successive birth cohorts so defined, the risk of congenital neural defects among military inductees clearly peaked in the birth cohort of October 15–December 31. A similar reanalysis of mortality data in these birth cohorts demonstrated that mortality related to CNS

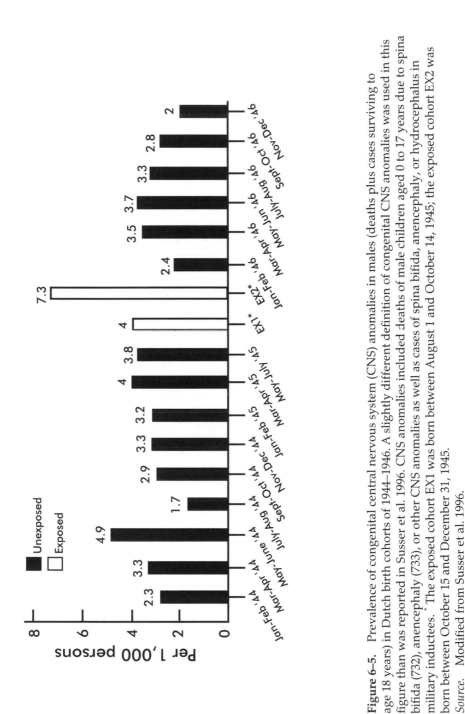

Figure 6–5. Prevalence of congenital central nervous system (CNS) anomalies in males (deaths plus cases surviving to age 18 years) in Dutch birth cohorts of 1944–1946. A slightly different definition of congenital CNS anomalies was used in this figure than was reported in Susser et al. 1996. CNS anomalies included deaths of male children aged 0 to 17 years due to spina bifida (733), anencephaly (732), or other CNS anomalies as well as cases of spina bifida, anencephaly, or hydrocephalus in military inductees. *The exposed cohort EX1 was born between August 1 and October 14, 1945; the exposed cohort EX2 was born between October 15 and December 31, 1945.
Source. Modified from Susser et al. 1996.

anomalies also peaked in the same cohort. Figure 6–5 shows the prevalence of congenital CNS anomalies in males, based on both the military induction data and the mortality data, in successive birth cohorts from 1944–1946.

Accordingly, the birth cohort of October 15–December 31, 1945, was defined as exposed to prenatal famine. All other birth cohorts of 1944–1946 in the cities of the famine region were defined as unexposed. Thus, exposed and unexposed birth cohorts were born only months apart in the same cities but differed in prenatal famine exposure.

Like the authors of the original Dutch Famine Study, we sought data sets that would enable us to determine the incidence of schizophrenia in exposed and unexposed birth cohorts without resorting to a costly follow-up of the individuals in these cohorts. The Dutch national psychiatric registry proved appropriate to this purpose. The registry data afforded comprehensive ascertainment of hospitalized schizophrenia in the exposed and unexposed birth cohorts. Registry data were available for 1970–1992. During this period, individuals in the birth cohorts of 1944–1946 were 24–48 years of age, well within the span of risk for schizophrenia. The registry encompassed admissions to psychiatric and university hospitals, which accounted for more than 90% of psychiatric admissions in The Netherlands. Data on each case included ICD Eighth/Ninth Revision (ICD-8/ICD-9; World Health Organization 1968, 1978) diagnosis as well as date and place of birth as required to define exposure.

We defined schizophrenia *a priori* to include only those cases in which the ICD-8/9 diagnosis was paranoid, hebephrenic, residual, or catatonic schizophrenia. This narrow definition of schizophrenia was in accordance with modern criteria for schizophrenia such as those in DSM-IV (American Psychiatric Association 1994) and ICD-10 (World Health Organization 1992). Although it severely restricted the number of cases, this definition also minimized the risk of misclassification of affective psychosis as schizophrenia.

The risk of schizophrenia was significantly increased in the exposed birth cohort (relative risk [RR] = 2.0) in both males (RR = 1.9) and females (RR = 2.2). Figure 6–6 shows the risk of schizophrenia in the same 17 successive birth cohorts of 1944–1946 that

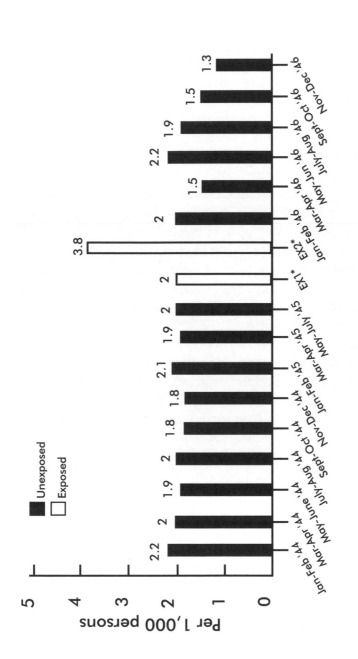

Figure 6–6. Risk of schizophrenia in adulthood in Dutch birth cohorts of 1944–1946: hospitalized cases in men and women 24–48 years of age. * The exposed cohort EX1 was born between August 1 and October 14, 1945; the exposed cohort EX2 was born between October 15 and December 31, 1945.
Source. Modified from Susser et al. 1996.

were used to illustrate the findings for congenital CNS anomalies in Figure 6–5. The risk of schizophrenia clearly peaked in the exposed cohort and was otherwise stable.

The remarkable coincidence in the peak of congenital CNS anomalies (Figure 6–5) and schizophrenia (Figure 6–6) in the exposed cohort is intriguing. The most compelling explanation for the excess in these disorders is early prenatal exposure to famine, which is well documented to have occurred only in the cohorts in which these disorders peaked.

Schizophrenia-Spectrum Personality Disorders

Genetic studies indicate that schizoid and schizotypal personality disorder are etiologically related to schizophrenia (Hoek and Kahn 1995; Kendler and Diehl 1993; Kendler et al. 1995; also see Chapter 2, this volume; Torgersen et al. 1993). Genes may confer a vulnerability that can be expressed in some cases as a personality disorder or some other related disorder and in other cases as schizophrenia. Similarly, it has been hypothesized that a prenatal brain insult may confer a vulnerability and be capable of a variety of manifestations. Some individuals may develop personality disorders and others schizophrenia, depending on the presence or absence of other exposures or genetic vulnerability.

For this reason, we extended our study of the Dutch famine cohorts to schizophrenia-spectrum personality disorders. We hypothesized that not only an increased risk of schizophrenia but also an increased risk of schizophrenia-spectrum personality disorders would be found among the birth cohorts that were conceived at the height of the famine and that showed an excess risk of schizophrenia at ages 24–48 years (Hoek et al. 1996).

For outcome data, we returned to the military induction data that were used in the original Dutch Famine Study. As described earlier, these data were available for all males at age 18 years in the exposed and the unexposed birth cohorts. The data included the ICD diagnosis of schizoid personality disorder based on the standardized military induction examination. Because the "schizotypal" diagnosis was not included in the ICD at that time, "schizoid personality" could include both schizoid and schizotypal personality disorders as defined in ICD-10/DSM-IV.

The ICD diagnoses of schizoid personality were made in accordance with ICD-8/9 guidelines (although recorded using ICD Sixth Revision [ICD-6; World Health Organization 1948] codes), which define schizoid personality as follows: "Personality disorder in which there is withdrawal from affectional, social and other contacts with autistic preference for fantasy and introspective reserve. Behavior may be slightly eccentric or indicate avoidance of competitive situations. Apparent coolness and detachment may mask an incapacity to express feeling" (World Health Organization 1978, p. 38). These criteria were interpreted restrictively by Dutch psychiatrists of the time, who used a narrow concept of schizoid personality disorder (Carp 1947; Rümke 1971).

We compared the prevalence of schizoid personality disorder in the military inductees of exposed and unexposed birth cohorts as defined previously in our schizophrenia study (Susser et al. 1996; Hoek et al. 1996). It should be noted that although the exposure data and the population were the same as in our schizophrenia study, the outcome data were collected independently. In addition, unlike the schizophrenia study, which relied on hospital registry data, these data were available for the entire male population, whether treated or untreated.

The exposed birth cohort had a significantly increased risk (RR = 2.01; 95% confidence interval [CI] = 1.03–3.94) of schizoid personality disorder compared with the unexposed cohorts. Moreover, as with congenital CNS anomalies and schizophrenia, the prevalence among birth cohorts of 1944–1946 clearly peaked in the exposed birth cohort (Figure 6–7).

All Schizophrenia-Spectrum Disorders

In a further analysis, we combined the cases of schizophrenia and of schizoid personality among males and examined the relationship of prenatal famine to all detectable schizophrenia-spectrum disorders among males (Hoek et al. 1998). This analysis required

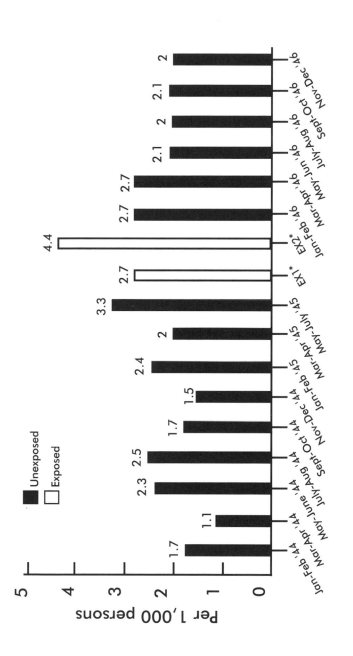

Figure 6–7. Prevalence of schizoid personality disorder after prenatal exposure to famine: male military inductees 18 years of age. * The exposed cohort EX1 was born between August 1 and October 14, 1945; the exposed cohort EX2 was born between October 15 and December 31, 1945.

Source. Modified from Hoek et al. 1996.

tracing the individual cases (Hoek et al. 1998) to determine overlap between the two case groups (otherwise, a case could be counted as schizoid at age 18 years and again as schizophrenia at ages 24–48 years).

The cases in the exposed birth cohort were traced, and the results revealed no overlap—that is, none of the cases in either of the two outcome data sets relate to the same person. At least in these cases, schizoid personality was not a precursor of hospitalized schizophrenia. Therefore, we could simply add the number of cases of each type for a combined analysis of the broader outcome of schizophrenia-spectrum disorders.

When this broader outcome was used, the peak in risk showed an even more precise association with prenatal famine exposure (Hoek et al. 1998). Thus, we found that the greatest increase in the risk of schizophrenia-spectrum disorders occurred among males born in the famine cities in December 1945 (RR = 2.7; 95% CI = 1.5–5.1). Individuals born in December 1945 were generally conceived at the absolute peak of the famine, in the last 8 weeks before the liberation in early May 1945.

New Research on Schizophrenia-Spectrum Disorders

While potentially illuminating, an association between prenatal famine and schizophrenia-spectrum disorders does not permit conclusions to be drawn regarding a causal mechanism. Our group has now embarked on a new program of research to elucidate the causal pathways (Hoek et al. 1998). This research entails tracing the individual famine-exposed case patients and conducting neurobiological studies in which these exposed patients are compared with unexposed patients and with exposed control subjects. Assessments include research diagnosis, course of illness, family/genetic history, analysis of genetic polymorphisms, neuroimaging, and minor physical anomalies.

The unique feature of this investigation is the uniform exposure to prenatal nutritional deficiency among the case patients of the exposed birth cohort. In light of the apparent heterogeneity of schizophrenia and of environmental exposures in a given population, traditional genetic linkage and association studies are not well suited to identify a genetic factor that operates via gene–environment interaction, that is, that requires the presence of a specific environmental factor to produce its effect (see Chapter 3, this volume). By examining a sample of case patients in which a large proportion share the same prenatal risk factor, however, it becomes possible to isolate a genetic factor that interacts with this prenatal factor. This feature also has implications for neurobiological studies. A sample of patients with the same prenatal exposure is likely to be enriched for certain etiologies of schizophrenia, facilitating detection of neurobiological correlates via magnetic resonance imaging and other assessments.

The investigation is still in progress, but we can describe its early phases. We began with 27 exposed schizophrenia case patients identified by the Dutch psychiatric registry. Among these, we were able to review the medical records for 20 patients. Medical records could not be reviewed for the other 7 patients because records were destroyed (2), lost (2), untraceable (1), or had duplicate registry numbers (2). Among the 20 for whom records were obtained, a thorough diagnostic review yielded a diagnosis of DSM-IV schizophrenia in 18 cases (90%), providing important support for the validity of the registry diagnoses used in the original report on schizophrenia (Susser et al. 1996). Assessments are currently being conducted with these case patients and with other spectrum case and control patients.

Pending the results of these investigations, we can speculate as to possible mechanisms, which fall into three general classes (Hoek et al. 1998).

First, general prenatal malnutrition could disrupt early brain development, thereby increasing vulnerability to schizophrenia-spectrum disorders. General malnutrition, which implies a gross deficiency of protein, calories, fat, or some combination of these, occurs mainly in developing countries and could be related to only a small number of cases of schizophrenia. Nonetheless, if this were shown to be the causal pathway, it would represent an important model, demonstrating that an early brain insult can have an impact on adult schizophrenia, and would likely lead to discovery of other related pathways.

Second, a highly specific prenatal micronutrient deficiency might be the key factor. Several other neurodevelopmental disorders have been related to specific prenatal nutrient deficiencies rather than to general malnutrition, and micronutrient deficiencies are well documented in developed as well as developing countries (Brown et al. 1996). Neural tube defects (NTDs), for instance, have been related to inadequate dietary folate in early gestation (Brown et al. 1996; Medical Research Council Vitamin Study Research Group 1991), and, like schizophrenia (Jablensky et al. 1992; Sartorius et al. 1986), NTDs are found in well-nourished as well as malnourished populations (Elwood et al. 1992). Indeed, we have speculated that the remarkable coincidence in timing between the peak in risk for schizophrenia and the peak in risk for congenital CNS anomalies—including NTDs—in the Dutch famine cohorts may be a clue that periconceptional folate deficiency also has relevance for schizophrenia (Susser et al. 1998b). NTDs are thought to result, in some cases, from a gene–environment interaction between a genetic defect in homocysteine metabolism and inadequate prenatal folate (van der Put et al. 1995; Whitehead et al. 1995). For this reason, we have been exploring the possibility that a genetic defect in homocysteine metabolism may play a role in schizophrenia (Susser et al. 1998b).

Third, a mediating factor might explain the observed association. The birth cohort with increased schizophrenia also had increased perinatal mortality, and there is evidence that perinatal complications are associated with an increased risk for schizophrenia. Yet, high perinatal mortality also affected some of the unexposed cohorts, which did not have elevated rates of schizophrenia. It has also been suggested that ingestion of tulip bulbs, which is reported to have occurred during the Hunger Winter, could have exerted a toxic effect on fetal brain development, or that hypersecretion of maternal corticosteroids may explain the observed effect. However, there is little solid evidence to support these alternative mechanisms.

New Research on the Full Spectrum of Psychosis

Our group has also initiated further studies to refine our understanding of the psychiatric outcome. This entails, in part, examining effects of prenatal exposure to the famine on the full range of nonaffective and affective psychosis. We have essentially employed the same research design model as for the studies of schizophrenia and schizoid personality disorder. Preliminary results indicate a significant increase in risk of paranoid psychosis (ICD-9 code 297) in the birth cohort exposed to the peak of the famine during the periconceptional period, consistent with the findings for schizophrenia and schizoid personality. Moreover, we have also demonstrated an increased risk of affective psychosis (ICD-9 code 296) in the birth cohorts exposed to the famine in the second and third trimesters (Brown et al. 1995). This finding raises the intriguing possibility that the nature and severity of the effect of prenatal famine on psychosis is related to the timing of the nutritional deficit during fetal development.

Conclusion

The Dutch Hunger Winter of 1944–1945 created a unique natural experiment that has been used to examine the relationship of prenatal famine to neurodevelopmental disorders, including schizophrenia. In studies of the Dutch famine cohorts, extending more than 30 years and over two generations of investigators, early prenatal famine has been found to be specifically and robustly associated with congenital anomalies of the CNS, schizophrenia, and schizophrenia-spectrum disorders (as well as with other health outcomes not discussed here [Lumey et al. 1998; G. P. Ravelli et al. 1976; A. C. J. Ravelli et al. 1998]). The results do not appear to be explained by selective conception or survival of exposed cases (Susser et al. 1998a) or by confounding due to social class (Susser et al. 1997), which was suggested by Van Os (1997).

In the belief that these associations may offer clues to the etiology of schizophrenia, we have undertaken a third generation of studies. These studies are guided by the hypothesis that prenatal micronutrient deficiencies can interact with genes to cause neuro-developmental schizophrenia. We hope to pursue this path of investigation until a specific etiology of neurodevelopmental schizophrenia can be established. Because prenatal micronutrient intake is easily modified by nutritional supplementation, the discovery of such an etiology would finally offer hope for the prevention of this devastating illness.

References

American Psychiatric Association: Diagnostic and Statistical Manual of Mental Disorders, 4th Edition. Washington, DC, American Psychiatric Association, 1994

Banning C: Food shortage and public health, first half of 1945. Annals of the American Academy of Political and Social Science 245:93–100, 1946

Bourne GH: Starvation in Europe. London, George Allen & Unwin, 1943

Breunis J: The food supply. Annals of the American Academy of Political and Social Science 245:87–92, 1946

Brown AS, Susser ES, Lin SP, et al: Increased risk of affective disorders in males after second trimester prenatal exposure to the Dutch Hunger Winter of 1944–45. Br J Psychiatry 166:601–606, 1995

Brown AS, Susser ES, Butler PD, et al: Neurobiological plausibility of prenatal nutritional deprivation as a risk factor for schizophrenia. J Nerv Ment Dis 184:71–85, 1996

Burger GCE, Drummond JC, Sandstead HR (eds): Malnutrition and Starvation in Western Netherlands: September 1944–July 1945. The Hague, General State Printing Office, 1948

Carp EADE: Medische Psychologie en Pathopsychologie. Amsterdam, Scheltema & Holkema, 1947

De Jong L: The Netherlands in the Second World War, Book 10, Part b: The Last Year. The Hague, Goverment Press, 1981

Dols MJL, van Arcken DJAM: Food supply and nutrition in The Netherlands during and after World War II. Milbank Memorial Fund Quarterly 24:319–355, 1946

Elwood JM, Little J, Elwood JH: Epidemiology and Control of Neural Tube Defects. New York, Oxford University Press, 1992

Hoek HW, Kahn RS: Genetic and environmental factors in the etiology of schizophrenia [Dutch: Erfelijkheid en omgevingsfactoren in de etiologie van schizofrenie]. Neth J Med 139:498–501, 1995

Hoek HW, Susser ES, Hulshof-Poll H, et al: Case–control and neuro-imaging study of schizophrenia after prenatal exposure to famine. Stanley Foundation Research Award, 1994

Hoek HW, Susser E, Buck KA, et al: Schizoid personality disorder after prenatal exposure to famine. Am J Psychiatry 153:1637–1639, 1996

Hoek HW, Brown AS, Susser E: The Dutch Famine and schizophrenia spectrum disorders. Soc Psychiatry Psychiatr Epidemiol (in press)

Jablensky A, Sartorius N, Ernberg G, et al: Schizophrenia: manifestations, incidence and course in different cultures: a World Health Organization 10-country study. Psychol Med Monogr Suppl 20:1–97, 1992

Kendler KS, Diehl SR: The genetics of schizophrenia: a current, genetic-epidemiologic perspective. Schizophr Bull 19:261–285, 1993

Kendler KS, Neale MC, Walsh D: Evaluating the spectrum concept of schizophrenia in the Roscommon study. Am J Psychiatry 152:749–754, 1995

Laurence KM, James N, Miller MH, et al: Double-blind randomized controlled trial of folate treatment before conception to prevent recurrence of neural tube defects. BMJ 282:1509–1511, 1981

Lumey LH, Stein AD: Offspring birthweights after maternal intrauterine undernutrition: a comparison within sibships. Am J Epidemiol 146:810–819, 1997

Medical Research Council Vitamin Study Research Group: Prevention of neural tube defects: results of the Medical Research Council Vitamin Study. Lancet 338:131–137, 1991

Mills JL, McPartlin JM, Kirke PN, et al: Homocysteine metabolism in pregnancies complicated by neural-tube defects. Lancet 345:149–151, 1995

Pasamanick B, Rogers ME, Lilienfeld AM: Pregnancy experience and the development of behavior disorder in children. Am J Psychiatry 112:613–618, 1956

Ravelli GP, Stein ZA, Susser MW: Obesity in young men after famine exposure in utero and early infancy. N Engl J Med 295:349–353, 1976

Ravelli ACJ, van der Meulen JHP, Michels RPJ, et al: Glucose tolerance in adults after prenatal exposure to famine. Lancet 351:173–177, 1998

Rümke HC: Psychiatrie. Amsterdam, Haarlem, Scheltema & Holkema NV, 1971

Sartorius N, Jablensky A, Korten G, et al: Early manifestations and first-contact incidence of schizophrenia in different cultures: a preliminary report on the initial evaluation of the WHO Collaborative Study on determinants of outcome of severe mental disorders. Psychol Med 16:909–928, 1986

Slager K, Feis N, van der Gaag P: Hunger Winter. Amsterdam, Link Publishers, 1985

Stein Z, Susser M, Saenger G, et al (eds): Famine and Human Development: The Dutch Hunger Winter of 1944–1945. New York, Oxford University Press, 1975

Susser ES, Lin SP: Schizophrenia after prenatal exposure to the Dutch Hunger Winter of 1944–45. Arch Gen Psychiatry 49:983–988, 1992

Susser ES, Neugebauer R, Hoek HW, et al: Schizophrenia after prenatal famine: further evidence. Arch Gen Psychiatry 53:25–31, 1996

Susser E, Neugebauer R, Hoek HW et al: Schizophrenia after prenatal famine (reply letter). Arch Gen Psychiatry 54:578, 1997

Susser E, Hoek HW, Brown A: Neurodevelopmental disorders after prenatal famine: the story of the Dutch Famine Study. Am J Epidemiol 147:213–216, 1998a

Susser E, Brown AS, Klonowski E, et al: Schizophrenia and impaired homocysteine metabolism: a possible association. Biol Psychiatry 44:141–143, 1998b

Torgersen S, Onstad S, Skre I, et al: "True" schizotypal personality disorder: a study of co-twins and relatives of schizophrenic probands. Am J Psychiatry 150:1661–1667, 1993

van der Put NMJ, Steegers-Theunissen RPM, Frosst P, et al: Mutated methylenetetrahydrofolate reductase as a risk factor for spina bifida. Lancet 346:1070–1071, 1995

Van Os J: Schizophrenia after prenatal famine. Arch Gen Psychiatry 54:577–578, 1997

Whitehead AS, Gallagher P, Mills JL, et al: A genetic defect in 5,10 methylenetetrahydrofolate reductase in neural tube defects. QJM 88:763–766, 1995

World Health Organization: International Classification of Diseases, Sixth Revision. Geneva, World Health Organization, 1948

World Health Organization: International Classification of Diseases, Eighth Revision. Geneva, World Health Organization, 1968

World Health Organization: Mental Disorders: Glossary and Guide to Their Classification in Accordance With the Ninth Revision of the International Classification of Diseases. Geneva, World Health Organization, 1978

World Health Organization: Mental Disorders: Glossary and Guide to Their Classification in Accordance With the Tenth Revision of the International Classification of Diseases. Geneva, World Health Organization, 1992

Chapter 7

Plausibility of Early Nutritional Deficiency as a Risk Factor for Schizophrenia

Pamela D. Butler, Ph.D., David Printz, M.D.,
Debbra Klugewicz, M.S., Alan S. Brown, M.D., and
Ezra S. Susser, M.D., Dr.P.H.

Since the 1950s, it has been hypothesized that prenatal nutritional deficiency is a risk factor in schizophrenia (Pasamanick et al. 1956). Recent findings by Susser and co-workers, demonstrating a twofold increase in risk of schizophrenia after exposure to famine during early gestation, have sparked renewed interest in this hypothesis (Susser and Lin 1992; Susser et al. 1996). Although these findings are intriguing, the hypothesis would be further supported by evidence that prenatal nutritional deficiency is neurobiologically plausible as a risk factor for schizophrenia.

The effects of prenatal nutritional deficiency as a cause of brain disorders in animals and humans have been well documented. However, the relevance of neurodevelopmental effects of prenatal nutritional depletion to schizophrenia has received scant attention in the literature.

The literature suggests that prenatal and postnatal protein and total calorie deprivation induces changes in brain function and structure that are relevant to brain alterations observed in schizophrenia. Early nutritional deprivation results in short- and long-term changes in neurotransmitter functioning, particularly of the serotonergic system; profound changes in brain morphology, especially of the hippocampus; and long-term changes in hippocampally mediated behaviors. Although more work remains to be done in this area, the likely importance of these brain regions and systems in the pathophysiology of schizophrenia supports the plausibility of early nutritional deficiency as a risk factor for this illness.

Thus, we begin this chapter by reviewing the effects of early nutritional deficiency on neurotransmitter functioning, brain morphology, and behavior in animal studies. We then discuss the potential relevance of these basic science (as opposed to clinical) studies to schizophrenia, noting the similarities in the effects of prenatal malnutrition on brain function and structure. For the sake of brevity, we limit our consideration to protein and total calorie deprivation. Specific prenatal micronutrient deficiencies that are believed to represent risk factors for schizophrenia, such as folate deficiency, have been reviewed elsewhere (Brown et al. 1996). It is hoped that this review will stimulate thinking about whether protein or total calorie deprivation constitutes a plausible candidate environmental risk factor for schizophrenia and suggest possible animal models for this illness.

General Review of Methodology

Before beginning our review of specific areas of study, we offer a note on the methodology of the studies presented. Protein deprivation and total calorie deprivation are two of the most widely studied models of nutritional deficiency. In protein-deprivation models, the pregnant rat is fed a diet that is restricted to protein only but otherwise isocaloric to the control diet. Protein-deprivation studies have generally either used an 8% or a 6% casein diet. Total-calorie-deprivation studies typically require a 50% restriction in caloric intake of the mother beginning at some time during gestation. For both types of studies, the period of undernutrition may be prenatal only, postnatal only, or both pre- and postnatal. Pups may be nutritionally rehabilitated at birth or at some point after weaning.

Neurotransmitter Functioning

We review the effects of early nutritional deficiency on seroto-nergic, dopaminergic, and noradrenergic functioning in two ways. First, we examine alterations in neurotransmitters during gestation and early development because neurotransmitters, particularly serotonin, affect neuronal growth and maturation (Huether 1990 [review]; Lauder and Bloom 1974; Olson and Seiger 1972). Second, we review the long-term effects of early nutritional deficiency on neurotransmitter functioning.

Early Developmental Effects

Protein-deprivation studies consistently show alterations of seroto-nergic systems (Table 7–1). Studies have examined the telencephalon and subtelencephalon in animals sacrificed at birth, and whole brain, telencephalon, diencephalon, midbrain, pons- medulla, and cerebellum in animals sacrificed in lactation and adulthood (Miller and Resnick 1980; Resnick and Morgane 1984).

Investigators have found activation of serotonergic systems following prenatal/postnatal protein deprivation, particularly in animals studied early in development (i.e., at birth or during lactation). Increased concentrations of serotonin and its metabolite 5-hydroxyindoleacetic acid (5-HIAA) were seen at birth (Stern et al. 1975) and during lactation (Miller and Resnick 1980; Miller et al. 1977; Resnick and Morgane 1984; Sobotka et al. 1974; Stern et al. 1975), suggesting increased serotonin turnover. The effects were seen after pre- plus postnatal protein deprivation as well as after prenatal protein deprivation alone. When animals are studied during lactation, studies also consistently show increased levels of the serotonin precursor tryptophan (Miller and Resnick 1980; Miller et al. 1977; Resnick and Morgane 1984) as well as increased levels of tryptophan hydroxylase, the rate-limiting enzyme in serotonin synthesis, following both prenatal and early postnatal protein deprivation (Miller and Resnick 1980). The increased concentrations of substrate and synthesizing enzyme may contribute to increased concentrations of serotonin.

Table 7–1. Neurotransmitter effects of prenatal and postnatal nutritional deprivation

Effect	Protein deprivation			Total calorie deprivation		
	Prenatal	Postnatal	Pre + Post	Prenatal	Postnatal	Pre + Post
DA						
DA levels	↔a↔b	↔f*↔r*	↔a↔o*			
DA turnover		↓p*	↓p*			
DA binding			↑i		↓t	
HVA levels	↔b	↔f*				
Tyrosine	↔b		↑c*↔o*↔p*			
Tyrosine hydroxylase			↑o*↑i			
NE						
NE levels	↑s**↔l* ↔c**↔a ↔b	↔r*	↑s↔c*↔i ↔a↓o*↓i* ↓l*↓p*		↔n*↔d*	
NE turnover			↑i↓p*		↓n	
NE binding			↓g		↓n*	
DHPG/MHPG levels	↔b	↔f*				
NE uptake			↔p*		↑n*	

Effect	Protein deprivation			Total calorie deprivation		
	Prenatal	Postnatal	Pre + Post	Prenatal	Postnatal	Pre + Post
5-HT						
5-HT levels	↑k*↑s** ↔l*↔c** ↔a↔b	↑*r↑k* ↓h	↑k*↑m*↑s* ↑j*↑s↔c* ↔a↓l*		↑d*↔d	
5-HT immunoreactive cell bodies and fibers					↓e*↓e	
5-HT synthesis					↑q	↑q
5-HT release	↑b					
5-HIAA levels	↑k*↑s** ↔b	↑*r↑k* ↓h	↑k*↑m*↑s* ↑j*↑s			
Tryptophan	↑k*↔b	↑k*↑o	↑k*↑m*↑j*			

Note. ↑ = increase; ↔ = no change; ↓ = decrease. DA = dopamine; HVA = homovanillic acid; NE = norepinephrine; 5-HT = 5-hydroxytryptamine (serotonin); 5-HIAA = 5-hydroxyindoleacetic acid; DHPG = dihydroxyphenylglycol; MHPG = methoxyhydroxyphenylglycol.

Studies: a = Ahmad and Rahman 1975; b = Chen et al. 1992; c = Dickerson and Pao 1975; d = Hernandez 1976; e = Ishimura et al. 1989; f = Juorio 1987; g = Keller et al. 1982; h = Klugewicz et al. 1995; i = Marichich et al. 1979; j = Miller et al. 1977; k = Miller and Resnick 1980; l = Ramanamurthy 1977; m = Resnick and Morgane 1984; n = Seidler et al. 1990; o = Shoemaker and Wurtman 1971; p = Shoemaker and Wurtman 1973; q = Smart et al. 1976; r = Sobotka et al. 1974; s = Stern et al. 1975; t = Wiggins et al. 1984. *Studied at birth. **Studied during lactation.

It is also important to note that several studies have showed no change (Ahmad and Rahman 1975; Dickerson and Pao 1975; Ramanamurthy 1977) or a decrease (Ramanamurthy 1977) in serotonin concentrations in animals sacrificed early in development. However, these studies examined whole brains, and thus changes in serotonin-rich brain areas may have been more difficult to detect. Thus, in the serotonergic system, at least when specific brain regions are examined, there are increased concentrations of serotonin as well as increased turnover.

In animals studied early in development, the effects of protein deprivation on norepinephrine and dopamine are less consistent than those on serotonin function (see Table 7–1). Unlike serotonin levels, which are consistently increased both at birth and during lactation, catecholamine levels may be either increased (Stern et al. 1975) or unchanged (Dickerson and Pao 1975; Ramanamurthy 1977) in animals sacrificed at birth and may be unchanged (Ahmad and Rahman 1975; Dickerson and Pao 1975; Juorio 1987; Sobotka et al. 1974) or decreased (Marichich et al. 1979; Ramanamurthy 1977; Shoemaker and Wurtman 1971, 1973) in animals studied during lactation. However, despite the general lack of increase in catecholamine concentrations following protein deprivation, it has been speculated (Marichich et al. 1979; Wiggins et al. 1984) that activation of noradrenergic and dopaminergic systems occurs because of increased concentrations of the catecholamine precursor tyrosine (Dickerson and Pao 1975 [but see Shoemaker and Wurtman 1971, 1973]); increased levels of tyrosine hydroxylase, the rate-limiting enzyme in catecholamine synthesis, have been found in rats studied early in development following protein deprivation (Shoemaker and Wurtman 1971). These results suggest increased turnover of catecholamines, although the findings are not yet definitive.

Long-Term Effects

Relatively few studies have examined the long-term consequences of early protein deprivation on serotonergic function (see Table 7–1), and findings are somewhat conflicting. Stern and colleagues (1975), examining all of the discrete brain regions mentioned previously, including midbrain and pons-medulla, found increased concentrations of serotonin and 5-HIAA, indicating activation of serotonergic systems into adulthood. However, Kohsaka and associates (1980), examining the brain stem as a whole, found no change in serotonin or 5-HIAA concentrations. Both of these studies used protein deprivation from gestation or lactation through adulthood. Thus, in the study of Stern et al. (1975), it is difficult to say whether early protein deprivation alone would have been sufficient to produce activation of serotonergic functioning that persisted until adulthood. Overall, while there is some evidence of long-term activation of serotonergic functioning following early protein deprivation, further investigation is needed.

Like results of studies of early development, findings regarding long-term effects of early protein deprivation on catecholamine functioning are inconsistent (see Table 7–1).

In conclusion, in animals examined early in development, serotonergic activation is the most consistent finding following early protein deprivation; the findings are particularly strong when specific brain regions are examined. Early effects of protein deficiency on dopamine and norepinephrine are less definitive. The literature is conflicting with respect to long-term increases in serotonin function and possible activation of catecholamine systems, but this area is also worthy of further exploration.

Relatively few studies have examined the effects of early total calorie deprivation on neurotransmitter functioning (for a review, see Table 7–1).

Brain Morphology

Studies of the effects of nutritional deficiency on brain morphology have particularly focused on the hippocampus (Table 7–2), abnormalities of which are frequently cited in imaging and postmortem studies of schizophrenia (Akbarian et al. 1993; Breier et al. 1992; Bogerts et al. 1990; Jakob and Beckmann 1986; Suddath et al. 1990; Waddington 1993). Prenatal malnutrition affects each part of the trisynaptic circuit of the hippocampus (Figure 7–1): The circuit's

Table 7–2. Morphological effects of prenatal and postnatal nutritional deprivation

	Protein deprivation			Total calorie deprivation		
Effect	Prenatal	Postnatal	Pre + Post	Prenatal	Postnatal	Pre + Post
Hippocampal formation						
Granule cells						
Cell number	↓i					↓a↓b↓c↓q
Cell size	↓i					↑a
Synapse/neuron ratio						
Number of synaptic spines			↓f			
Number of dendritic spines			↓f			
Dendritic branching						
Granule layer thickness						↓t*
Granule cell layer volume						↔c
Cell acquisition rate						↓t*
Cell cycle time						↑t*
Length of S phase						↑t*
Length of G_2 phase						↑t*
Length of G_1 phase						↓t*
Neurogenesis	↓h					

Effect	Protein deprivation			Total calorie deprivation		
	Prenatal	Postnatal	Pre + Post	Prenatal	Postnatal	Pre + Post
Pyramidal cells						
CA3 cell number						↓q
CA4 cell number						↓q
Somal size	↓m		↓p			
Dendritic branching	↓m		↓p			
Dendritic diameter	↓m		↓p			
General						
Thickness						↓r
DNA					↓o*	
Protein					↓o*	
Protein/DNA ratio					↔o*	
Cortex						
Cerebrum						
Weight					↓r	↓r
Length					↓r	↓r
Width					↓r	↓r
Thickness						↓r

(continued)

Table 7–2. Morphological effects of prenatal and postnatal nutritional deprivation (*continued*)

Effect	Protein deprivation			Total calorie deprivation		
	Prenatal	Postnatal	Pre + Post	Prenatal	Postnatal	Pre + Post
Cortex (*continued*)						
Cerebrum (continued)						
DNA content					$\downarrow$o*	
Protein content					$\downarrow$o*	
Protein/DNA ratio					$\downarrow$o*	
Cortical neurons						
Cell number						$\leftrightarrow$e
Visual cortex						
Changes in complexity of dendrites of pyramidal neurons						1
Forebrain						
Ventricular subependymal layer						
Cell cycle time						$\uparrow$s
Length of S phase						$\uparrow$s
Length of G_2 phase						$\leftrightarrow$s
Length of G_1 phase						$\uparrow$s

Effect	Protein deprivation			Total calorie deprivation		
	Prenatal	Postnatal	Pre + Post	Prenatal	Postnatal	Pre + Post
Cell acquisition						↓s
Cell degeneration						↑s
Forebrain/weight ratio						↓a
Cell migration						
Rate from anterior lateral ventricle to olfactory bulb		↓g				
Limbic system						
Fornix						
Cell number						↓q
Medial septum						
Cell number						↓q
Amygdaloid nuclear complex						
Dendritic area					↓n	
Somatic area					↓n	

(continued)

Table 7–2. Morphological effects of prenatal and postnatal nutritional deprivation (*continued*)

Effect	Protein deprivation			Total calorie deprivation		
	Prenatal	Postnatal	Pre + Post	Prenatal	Postnatal	Pre + Post
Brain stem						
DNA content					↓o*	
Protein content					↓o*	
Protein/DNA ratio					↓o*	
Nucleus raphe dorsalis						
Lack of normal age-related changes in dendritic spine density		↓j*				
Locus coeruleus						
Lack of normal age-related changes in dendritic spine density		↓k*				
Cerebellum						
Purkinje cell numbers					↔d	↓d
DNA content					↓o*	
Protein content					↓o*	

Effect	Protein deprivation			Total calorie deprivation		
	Prenatal	Postnatal	Pre + Post	Prenatal	Postnatal	Pre + Post
Protein/DNA ratio					↔o*	
Weight						↓u
Synapse/neuron ratio						↓u
Whole brain						
DNA content					↓o*	
Protein content					↓o*	
Protein/DNA ratio					↓o*	
Weight					↓n	

Note. ↑ = increase; ↔ = no change; ↓ = decrease. DA = dopamine; HVA = homovanillic acid; NE = norepinephrine; 5-HT = 5-hydroxytryptamine (serotonin); 5-HIAA = 5-hydroxyindoleacetic acid; DHPG = dihydroxyphenylglycol; MHPG = methoxyhydroxyphenylglycol.

Studies: a = Ahmed et al. 1987; b = Bedi 1991a; c = Bedi 1991b; d = Bedi 1994; e = Bedi et al. 1992; f = Cintra et al. 1990; g = Debassio and Kemper 1985; h = Debassio et al. 1994; i = Diaz-Cintra et al. 1981; j = Diaz-Cintra et al. 1984; k = Diaz-Cintra et al. 1990; l = Diaz-Cintra et al. 1991; m = Diaz-Cintra et al. 1994; n = Escobar and Salas 1993; o = Fish and Winick 1969; p = Garcia-Ruiz et al. 1993; q = Jordan et al. 1982; r = Katz et al. 1982; s = Lewis et al. 1977; t = Lewis et al. 1979; u = Warren MA, Bedi 1990.

*Studied during lactation.

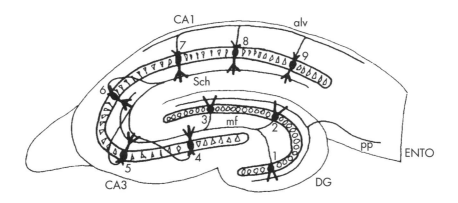

Figure 7–1. Hippocampal trisynaptic circuit. alv = alveus; DG = dentate gyrus; ENTO = entorhinal cortex; mf = mossy fibers; pp = perforant path; Sch = Schaffer collaterals.
Source. Reprinted from Teyler TJ, DiScenna P: "The Topological Anatomy of the Hippocampus: A Clue to Its Function." *Brain Research Bulletin* 12:713, 1984, with kind permission of Elsevier Science   NL, Sara Burgerhartstraat 25, 1055 KV Amsterdam, The Netherlands.

three parts consist of 1) perforant pathway input to hippocampal dentate granule cells, 2) granule cell input to CA3 pyramidal cells via mossy fibers, and 3) CA3 input to CA1 pyramidal cells via Schaffer collaterals. Axons of CA1 pyramidal cells exit the hippocampus via the alveus (for a review, see Teyler and DiScenna 1984).

Protein Deprivation

A number of basic science studies have examined the effects of protein deprivation on hippocampal morphology (see Table 7–2). Protein deprivation during gestation and up to the time of sacrifice at 30, 90, or 220 days caused decreases in terminal dendritic branching of dentate granule cell apical dendrites in the molecular layer and also produced a significant reduction in the number of dendritic spines in the outer two-thirds of these apical dendrites (Cintra et al. 1990).

An important question that arises is the timing of these teratogenic effects. In the rat, it is known that neurogenesis of hippocampal granule cells takes place primarily during the first 25 days after birth. Dobbing and co-workers (Dobbing 1981; Smart and Dobbing 1971) have argued that the rodent brain is spared from nutritional deprivation during gestation. However, Morgane and associates (1993) reported that prenatal nutritional deprivation can alter postnatal neurogenesis. They hypothesized that the prenatal period is a critical time in producing long-term alterations in hippocampal morphology, so that protein deprivation during this time would have profound effects. Consistent with this assertion, Diaz-Cintra and colleagues (1991) found altered hippocampal granule cell apical dendrites in mature rat brains when protein deprivation was restricted to the prenatal period and followed by dietary rehabilitation at birth.

Similar morphological changes occur in hippocampal CA3 pyramidal cells, which receive input from the granule cells via mossy fibers. Protein deprivation of rats during gestation and until sacrifice at 30, 90, or 220 days has been demonstrated to result in decreased somal size of CA3 pyramidal cells at 220 days, decreased diameter of apical dendrites at 30 and 90 days, and decreased branching of the outer third of apical dendrites at 220 days (Garcia-Ruiz et al. 1993); similar changes occurred when protein deficiency was restricted to the prenatal period (Diaz-Cintra et al. 1994).

Thus, in terms of hippocampal development, protein deprivation during the prenatal period only, which roughly corresponds to the first half of gestation in humans, is sufficient to alter development in long-lasting ways.

Other brain areas are also affected by protein deprivation. For instance, rats deprived of protein from gestation until adulthood showed age-related changes in dendritic complexity of pyramidal neurons in the visual cortex, in contrast to control rats (Diaz-Cintra et al. 1990). Brain-stem serotonergic and noradrenergic areas are also affected (see Table 7–2). Neurons in the brain-stem nucleus raphe dorsalis, which contains the majority of central nervous system (CNS) serotonin cell bodies, and the nucleus locus coeruleus, the major norepinephrine-containing nucleus in the CNS, do not show the increases in dendritic spine density normally observed between early development and adulthood in animals subjected to protein deprivation beginning in gestation and continuing until sacrifice at 30, 90, or 220 days (Diaz-Cintra et al. 1981, 1984).

Several studies have begun to explore the reasons for the altered morphology seen in protein-deprived rats. For example, DeBassio and Kemper (1985) found that rats protein-deprived from gestation until sacrifice shortly after weaning had slower migration of neurons from the anterior lateral ventricle to the olfactory bulb. Slower migration of neurons early in development may be related to abnormalities of cell differentiation seen later on because normal maturation may rely on the sequential and timely arrival of neurons at their appropriate places in the CNS. A more recent study by DeBassio and colleagues (1994) showed decreased prenatal neurogenesis of granule cells, but not pyramidal cells, in prenatally protein-deprived rats. This finding is of interest because decreased granule cell genesis could potentially contribute to altered granule cell morphology seen in adulthood.

We have recently found preliminary evidence of increased basal corticosterone levels in prenatally protein-deprived animals that were studied in adulthood (Butler et al. 1995). Because of the role of corticosterone in granule cell neurogenesis and cell death (Gould et al. 1991a, 1991b), it would be important to determine whether there are increased levels of corticosterone in the first few weeks of life following early protein deprivation.

Total Calorie Deprivation

A number of basic science studies have examined the effects of total calorie deprivation on hippocampal morphology (see Table 7–2). Total calorie deprivation during gestation and lactation consistently produces decreases in granule cell number in the dentate gyrus in adult rats (Ahmed et al. 1987; Bedi 1991a, 1991b; Jordan et al. 1982). These decreases could impair the ability of granule cells to appropriately gate incoming information from the perforant path. There are also decreased numbers of CA3 and CA1 pyramidal cells (Jordan et al. 1982), and this could alter the flow of information within the hippocampus and the output via the alveus, respectively. Alterations are likewise seen in the cerebral cortex, limbic system, brain stem, cerebellum, and whole brain (see Table 7–2).

Behavioral Changes

Morphological studies demonstrating hippocampal damage and biochemical studies showing altered serotonergic and catecholaminergic functioning suggest that early nutritional deprivation may affect behavior, particularly those aspects associated with neurotransmitter and hippocampal function.

Whereas few studies have examined serotonin- or catecholamine-mediated behaviors in rats subjected to early nutritional deprivation, a number of studies have examined hippocampally mediated behaviors in animals subjected to protein or total calorie deprivation. In rats, the hippocampus is involved in the ability to monitor spatial location (Olton and Samuelson 1976) as well as in learning and memory (Randt and Derby 1973), including working memory (Kitajima et al. 1992; Olton et al. 1979). Indeed, hippocampal damage may underlie deficits in learning and memory seen after early damage to the nervous system (Randt and Derby 1973).

Protein Deprivation

Tonkiss and co-workers studied rats that had been prenatally deprived of protein and subsequently nutritionally rehabilitated until adulthood. These animals showed deficits on a number of hippocampally mediated behaviors (Table 7–3). The deficits included more errors and longer time to reach criteria on a visual discrimination task (Tonkiss et al. 1991b), impaired ability to learn a task that required withholding responses (Tonkiss et al. 1990), and increased resistance to extinction on a food-rewarded alternation task with an elevated T-maze (Tonkiss and Galler 1990). However, not all hippocampally related behaviors were affected; prenatally protein-deprived animals did not show deficits on a working memory task that used delayed alternation, which involves the hippocampus (Tonkiss and Galler 1990), or in the partial reinforcement extinction effect (Tonkiss et al. 1991a).

A series of studies by Lipska and co-workers (Lipska and Weinberger 1993; Lipska et al. 1993) demonstrated that neonatal lesions of the ventral hippocampus produced increased dopamine-mediated locomotion and stereotypy. We have hypothesized (Butler et al. 1994) that prenatal protein deprivation, which also alters hippocampal morphology (see section titled "Brain Morphology," above), may produce changes in dopamine-mediated behaviors. In beginning to examine this question, we have recently found increases in dopamine-mediated stereotypy and locomotion in adult rats following prenatal protein deprivation, although catalepsy was not altered (Klugewicz et al. 1995).

Therefore, prenatal protein deprivation produces behavioral deficits in a number of hippocampally mediated behaviors and in some dopamine-mediated behaviors in rats.

Total Calorie Deprivation

Studies of total calorie deprivation have also focused on hippocampally mediated behaviors. In these studies, unlike protein deprivation studies, nutritional deprivation included gestation, gestation plus lactation, or lactation only. The findings indicate that behavioral deficits tend to occur in adulthood only when nutritional deprivation included the prenatal period. For instance, animals receiving 50% calorie deprivation during gestation showed deficits in their ability to choose the correct arm of a maze on a visual discrimination task (Jaiswal and Bhattacharya 1993). Animals receiving 50% calorie deprivation during both gestation and lactation had altered spatial learning ability, as manifested by increased time to make choices in a maze and decreased exploration of a novel environment (Jordan et al. 1981), and failed to exhibit spontaneous alternation (Jordan et al. 1982). Of particular interest is the finding that abolition of spontaneous alternation was correlated with reduced cell count in the hippocampus (Jordan et al. 1982).

When nutritional deprivation was restricted to the lactation period, no deficits were found in hippocampally mediated behaviors in adulthood, including spatial memory (Slob et al. 1973) and escape acquisition in a water maze (Campbell and Bedi 1989; Castro et al. 1989).

A final point worth considering is the timing of nutritional rehabilitation in relation to behavioral deficits. Two studies found that

Table 7–3. Behavioral effects of prenatal and postnatal nutritional deprivation

Effect	Protein deprivation			Total calorie deprivation		
	Prenatal	Postnatal	Pre + Post	Prenatal	Postnatal	Pre + Post
Spatial learning and memory	↔o ↔o*		↓e ↔e	↓g	↓d* ↓c ↓d ↔j ↔d ↔b	↓a* ↓h ↓i ↔f ↔a
Visual learning and memory	↓n				↔j	
Working memory	↔k					
Other types of learning and memory	↓l				↓d	
Extinction	↔m ↓k					

Note. ↔ = no change; ↓ = decrease. DA = dopamine; HVA = homovanillic acid; NE = norepinephrine; 5-HT = 5-hydroxytryptamine (serotonin); 5-HIAA = 5-hydroxyindoleacetic acid; DHPG = dihydroxyphenylglycol; MHPG = methoxyhydroxyphenylglycol.
Studies: a = Bedi 1992; b = Campbell and Bedi 1989; c = Castro and Rudy 1987; d = Castro et al. 1989; e = Goodlett et al. 1986; f = Hall 1983; g = Jaiswal and Bhattacharya 1993; h = Jordan et al. 1981; i = Jordan et al. 1982; j = Slob et al. 1973; k = Tonkiss and Galler 1990; l = Tonkiss et al. 1990; m = Tonkiss et al. 1991a; n = Tonkiss et al. 1991b; o = Tonkiss et al. 1994.
*Studied during lactation.

deficits are more likely to occur at the beginning of nutritional rehabilitation than after longer periods of nutritional rehabilitation. Decreased escape acquisition in a water maze was found when testing occurred immediately after the start of nutritional rehabilitation at the end of lactation, but no maze-learning deficit was observed when testing occurred after nutritional rehabilitation until adulthood (Bedi 1992; Castro et al. 1989). Thus, there may be a significant recovery of function in pathways required for those tasks.

Relevance of Basic Science Studies to Schizophrenia

Basic science studies consistently show that early protein and total calorie deprivation affect the CNS, particularly neurotransmitter function, hippocampal morphology, and hippocampal and possibly dopamine-mediated behaviors. These findings are relevant to schizophrenia, in which disruptions of neurotransmitter function and structural abnormalities of the hippocampus have been repeatedly found (Bogerts et al. 1990; Davis et al. 1991; Liddle et al. 1992; Meltzer 1989; Musalek et al. 1989; Suddath et al. 1990).

Neurotransmitter Abnormalities

Parallel to findings of increased serotonin and catecholamine activity in adult rats after prenatal protein deprivation, patients with schizophrenia also demonstrate abnormalities in these neurotransmitter systems; for each, excessive activity has been postulated. In schizophrenia, the findings appear strongest for dopamine and serotonin (Davis et al. 1991; Joyce 1993; Kahn and Davis 1995; Meltzer 1989; Roth and Meltzer 1995), although noradrenergic dysfunction has also been observed (van Kammen et al. 1989). Continued work since the inception of the "dopamine hypothesis" suggests a defect of plastic adaptive functioning of dopamine systems in schizophrenia (Friedhoff 1986, 1988; Grace 1991). The role of serotonin in schizophrenia is also of interest, because new, clinically effective atypical antipsychotic drugs, such as clozapine and risperidone, have serotonin$_{2A}$-blocking activity (Meltzer 1995).

These findings are also of relevance when viewed within the context of the neurodevelopmental hypothesis of schizophrenia. A growing literature supports a disturbance of brain development in the etiopathogenesis of schizophrenia (Murray and Lewis 1987; Waddington 1993; Weinberger 1987) and suggests a disruption of neuronal migration (Akbarian et al. 1993; Kovelman and Scheibel 1984). Serotonin, dopamine, and norepinephrine have each been shown to alter neuronal migration. For instance, at high levels, serotonin has an inhibitory effect on cell migration and may regulate cell migration by binding to receptors or to components of the extracellular matrix (for a review, see Lauder 1993). Catecholamines may also be important in cell migration, given that neonatal administration of 6-hydroxydopamine, which depletes catecholamines, causes decreases in cerebellar granule cell migration and number, abnormal foliation, fissuration, disorientation of Purkinje dendritic trees in the cerebellum (for a review, see Lauder and Krebs 1984), and abnormalities of cell migration in the cerebral cortex (Lidov and Molliver 1979). Thus, it is conceivable that prenatal protein and calorie malnutrition might lead to schizophrenia through two mechanisms, one involving a prenatal developmental disturbance and the other involving pathophysiological effects of neurotransmitter dysfunction in adulthood.

Brain Morphological Abnormalities

There are several similarities between brain morphological changes observed following prenatal protein and calorie deprivation and structural abnormalities found in schizophrenia. As previously discussed, abnormalities of hippocampal granule and pyramidal cell populations are present after prenatal protein and total calorie deprivation and have also been demonstrated in patients with schizophrenia. In addition to diminished hippocampal size, observed in imaging studies in schizophrenic patients (Bogerts et al. 1993; Breier et al. 1992), postmortem studies of the dentate gyrus have shown decreased depth (McLardy 1974), volume, and cell number in the hippocampus (Falkai and Bogerts 1986; Falkai et al. 1988). In another postmortem study, Goldsmith and Joyce (1995) found decreased density of mossy fibers, which are the axons of granule cells that innervate CA3 pyramidal cells. Limbic and cortical areas are also altered in nutritionally deprived animals, findings with potential relevance to postmortem studies of schizophrenia, which have found abnormal cell densities, patterns, and volumes in various regions including cortex and limbic system (Akbarian et al. 1993; Bogerts et al. 1990; Jakob and Beckmann 1986; Suddath et al. 1990).

It has been postulated that reduced cell densities and volumes in a number of brain regions investigated in the brains of patients with schizophrenia reflect a failure of proliferation/migration or excessive neuronal dropout early in life, possibly during fetal or neonatal development (Akbarian et al. 1993; Bogerts et al. 1990; Cannon and Mednick 1991). This lends credibility to prenatal and early postnatal nutritional deprivation as a risk factor in the structural abnormalities associated with a neurodevelopmental model of schizophrenia.

Behavioral Abnormalities

The finding of deficits in hippocampally mediated behaviors related to learning and memory in animals following early nutritional deprivation has relevance for schizophrenia, given that cognitive deficits, including memory dysfunction (especially for working memory) and inability to "tune out" (gate) irrelevant incoming stimuli, have been repeatedly found in patients with schizophrenia (Gur et al. 1994; for a review, see Venables 1992). In addition, as reviewed above, a number of brain-imaging and postmortem studies have shown hippocampal damage in patients with schizophrenia.

Conclusion

In this chapter we have demonstrated that protein and calorie deprivation early in development causes morphological, neurotransmitter, and behavioral changes that bear intriguing similarities to neuropathological and neurocognitive findings in schizophrenia.

As reviewed by Hoek and colleagues in Chapter 6, epidemiological studies indicate that prenatal nutritional deprivation is a potential risk factor for schizophrenia. Thus, the findings reviewed in this chapter, including our recent findings of increased dopamine-mediated behaviors in adulthood, as well as increased corticosterone levels, in prenatally protein-deprived adult rats (Butler et al. 1995; Klugewicz et al. 1995) parallel some aspects of the neuropathology of schizophrenia and could be used in future work to develop an animal model of relevance to schizophrenia. In tandem with epidemiological studies in humans, our laboratory is examining whether prenatal protein deprivation affects granule cell neurogenesis during the first few weeks of life. Examining the effects of early nutritional deficiency on neurogenesis, migration, and cell death could lead to a better understanding of the developmental sequelae of events that lead to altered brain morphology and function in both schizophrenia and normal adulthood. We are also investigating whether corticosterone, which acts as a morphogenetic signal early in life, might be increased in the first few weeks of life by early nutritional deficiency and thus might contribute to altered brain morphology. Similarly, it would be of interest to determine whether serotonin, which also acts as a morphogenetic signal early in life and is known to be altered by early nutritional deficiency, plays a role in abnormal brain morphology.

Moreover, this animal model promises to enable investigators to examine the neuropathological, neurochemical, and behavioral effects of specific nutritional deficiencies that have been implicated as risk factors for schizophrenia. For example, neurodevelopmental effects of prenatal deficiencies of micronutrients, such as folic acid, could be examined via this paradigm. In addition, these types of studies could have profound implications for elucidating the pathogenic mechanisms of these nutritional deficiencies as causes of brain developmental disturbances. Finally, since genetic models of neurodevelopmental disorders such as neural tube defects already exist, preclinical studies on interactions between genes and prenatal nutrition (see Chapter 2, this volume) have the potential to complement our epidemiological investigations in this area. Through this dynamic and unique interplay between the basic and the clinical sciences, we expect to move ever closer toward solving the etiological puzzle of schizophrenia.

References

Ahmad G, Rahman MA: Effects of undernutrition and protein malnutrition on brain chemistry of rats. J Nutr 105:1090–1103, 1975

Ahmed MGE, Bedi KS, Warren MA, et al: Effects of a lengthy period of undernutrition from birth and subsequent nutritional rehabilitation on the synapse: granule cell neuron ratio in the rat dentate gyrus. J Comp Neurol 263:146–158, 1987

Akbarian S, Vinuela A, Kim JJ, et al: Distorted distribution of nicotinamide-adenine dinucleotide phosphate-diaphorase neurons in temporal lobe of schizophrenics implies anomalous cortical development. Arch Gen Psychiatry 50:178–187, 1993

Bedi KS: Effects of undernutrition during early life on granule cell numbers in the rat dentate gyrus. J Comp Neurol 311:425–433, 1991a

Bedi KS: Early life undernutrition causes deficits in rat dentate gyrus granule cell number. Experientia 47:1073–1074, 1991b

Bedi KS: Spatial learning ability of rats undernourished during early postnatal life. Physiol Behav 51:1001–1007, 1992

Bedi KS: Undernutrition of rats during early life does not affect the total number of cortical neurons. J Comp Neurol 342:596–602, 1994

Bedi KS, Campbell LF, Mayhew TM: A fractionator study of the effects of undernutrition during early life on rat Purkinje cell numbers (with a caveat on the use of nucleoli as counting units). J Anat 181:199–208, 1992

Bogerts B, Ashtari M, Degreef G, et al: Reduced temporal limbic structure volumes on magnetic resonance images in first-episode schizophrenia. Psychiatry Res 35:1–13, 1990

Bogerts B, Lieberman JA, Ashtari M, et al: Hippocampus-amygdala volumes and psychopathology in chronic schizophrenia. Biol Psychiatry 33:236–246, 1993

Breier A, Buchanan RW, Elkashef A, et al: Brain morphology and schizophrenia: a magnetic resonance imaging study of limbic, prefrontal cortex, and caudate structures. Arch Gen Psychiatry 49:921–926, 1992

Brown AS, Susser ES, Butler PD, et al: Neurobiological plausibility of prenatal nutritional deprivation as a risk factor for schizophrenia. J Nerv Ment Dis 184:71–85, 1996

Butler PD, Susser ES, Brown AS, et al: Prenatal nutritional deprivation as a risk factor in schizophrenia: preclinical evidence. Neuropsychopharmacology 11:227–235, 1994

Butler PD, Klugewicz DA, Ciplet D, et al: Effects of prenatal protein deprivation on corticosterone levels in adult rats. Society for Neuroscience Abstracts 21:2015, 1995

Campbell LF, Bedi KS: The effects of undernutrition during early life on spatial learning. Physiol Behav 45:883–890, 1989

Cannon TD, Mednick SA: Fetal neural development and adult schizophrenia: an elaboration of the paradigm, in Fetal Neural Development and Adult Schizophrenia. Edited by Mednick SA, Cannon TD, Barr CE, et al. New York, Cambridge University Press, 1991, pp 227–237

Castro CA, Rudy JR: Early-life malnutrition selectively retards the development of distal but not proximal-cue navigation. Dev Psychobiol 20:521–537, 1987

Castro CA, Tracy M, Rudy JR: Early life undernutrition impairs the development of learning and short-term memory processes mediating performance in a conditional-spatial discrimination task. Behav Brain Res 32:255–264, 1989

Chen JC, Tonkiss J, Galler JR, et al: Prenatal protein malnutrition in rats enhances serotonin release from hippocampus. J Nutr 122:2138–2143, 1992

Cintra L, Diaz-Cintra S, Galvan A, et al: Effects of protein undernutrition on the dentate gyrus in rats of three age groups. Brain Res 532:271–277, 1990

Davis KL, Kahn RS, Ko G, et al: Dopamine in schizophrenia: a review and reconceptualization. Am J Psychiatry 148:1474–1486, 1991

Debassio WA, Kemper TL: The effects of protein deprivation on neuronal migration in rats. Developmental Brain Research 20:191–196, 1985

Debassio WA, Kemper TL, Galler JR, et al: Prenatal malnutrition effect on pyramidal and granule cell generation in the hippocampal formation. Brain Res Bull 35:57–61, 1994

Diaz-Cintra S, Cintra L, Kemper T, et al: The effects of protein deprivation on the nucleus raphe dorsalis: a morphometric Golgi study in rats of three age groups. Brain Res 221:243–255, 1981

Diaz-Cintra S, Cintra L, Kemper T, et al: The effects of protein deprivation on the nucleus locus coeruleus: a morphometric Golgi study in rats of three age groups. Brain Res 304:243–253, 1984

Diaz-Cintra S, Cintra L, Ortega A, et al: Effects of protein deprivation on pyramidal cells of the visual cortex in rats of three age groups. J Comp Neurol 292:117–126, 1990

Diaz-Cintra S, Cintra L, Galvan A, et al: Effects of prenatal protein deprivation on postnatal development of granule cells in the fascia dentata. J Comp Neurol 310:356–364, 1991

Diaz-Cintra S, Garcia-Ruiz M, Corkidi G, et al: Effects of prenatal malnutrition and postnatal nutritional rehabilitation on CA3 hippocampal pyramidal cells in rats of four ages. Brain Res 662:117–126, 1994

Dickerson JWT, Pao SK: Effect of pre- and post-natal maternal protein deficiency on free amino acids and amines of rat brain. Biol Neonate 25: 114–124, 1975

Dobbing J: The later development of the brain and its vulnerability, in Scientific Foundations of Pediatrics. Edited by Davis JA, Dobbing J. London, Heinemann Medical Books, 1981, pp 744–757

Escobar C, Salas M: Neonatal undernutrition and amygdaloid nuclear complex development: an experimental study in the rat. Exp Neurol 122:311–318, 1993

Falkai P, Bogerts B: Cell loss in the hippocampus of schizophrenics. European Archives of Psychiatry and Neurological Sciences 236:154–161, 1986

Falkai P, Bogerts B, Rozumek M: Limbic pathology in schizophrenia: the entorhinal region—a morphogenetic study. Biol Psychiatry 24:515–521, 1988

Fish I, Winick M: Effect of malnutrition on regional growth of the developing rat brain. Exp Neurol 25:534–540, 1969

Friedhoff AJ: A dopamine-dependent restitutive system for the maintenance of mental normalcy. Ann N Y Acad Sci 463:47–52, 1986

Friedhoff AJ: Adaptation of the dopaminergic system in the pathophysiology and treatment of schizophrenia. Psychopharmacol Bull 24: 335–337, 1988

Garcia-Ruiz M, Diaz-Cintra S, Cintra L, et al: Effect of protein malnutrition on CA3 hippocampal pyramidal cells in rats of three ages. Brain Res 625:203–212, 1993

Goldsmith SK, Joyce JN: Alterations in hippocampal mossy fiber pathway in schizophrenia and Alzheimer's disease. Biol Psychiatry 37:122–126, 1995

Goodlett CR, Valentino ML, Morgane PJ, et al: Spatial cue utilization in chronically malnourished rats: task specific learning deficits. Dev Psychobiol 19:1–15, 1986

Gould E, Woolley CS, Cameron HA, et al: Adrenal steroids regulate postnatal development of the rat dentate gyrus, II: effects of gluco-corticoids and mineralocorticoids on cell birth. J Comp Neurol 313: 486–493, 1991a

Gould E, Woolley CS, McEwen BS: Adrenal steroids regulate postnatal development of the rat dentate gyrus, I: effects of glucocorticoids on cell death. J Comp Neurol 313:479–485, 1991b

Grace AA: Phasic versus tonic dopamine release and the modulation of dopamine system responsivity: a hypothesis for the etiology of schizophrenia. Neuroscience 41:1–24, 1991

Gur RE, Jaggi JL, Shtasel DL, et al: Cerebral blood flow in schizophrenia: effects of memory processing on regional activation. Biol Psychiatry 35:3–15, 1994

Hall R: Is hippocampal function in the adult rat impaired by early protein or protein-calorie deficiencies? Dev Psychobiol 16:395–411, 1983

Hernandez RJ: Effects of malnutrition and 6-hydroxydopamine on the early postnatal development of noradrenaline and serotonin content in the rat brain. Biol Neonate 30:181–186, 1976

Huether G: Malnutrition and developing synaptic transmitter systems: lasting effects, functional implications, in (Mal)nutrition and the Infant Brain. Edited by Van Gelder NM, Butterworth RF, Drujan BD. New York, Wiley-Liss, 1990, pp 141–156

Ishimura K, Takeuchi Y, Fujiwara K, et al: Effects of undernutrition on the serotonin neuron system in the developing brain: an immunohistochemical study. Dev Brain Res 50:225–231, 1989

Jaiswal AK, Bhattacharya SK: Effect of gestational undernutrition, stress and diazepam treatment on spatial discrimination learning and retention in young rats. Indian J Exp Biol 31:353–359, 1993

Jakob H, Beckmann H: Prenatal developmental disturbances in the limbic allocortex in schizophrenics. J Neural Transm 65:303–326, 1986

Jordan TC, Cane SE, Howells KF: Deficits in spatial memory performance induced by early undernutrition. Dev Psychobiol 14:317–325, 1981

Jordan TC, Howells KF, McNaughton N, et al: Effects of early undernutrition on hippocampal development and function. Res Exp Med (Berl) 180:201–207, 1982

Joyce JN: The dopamine hypothesis of schizophrenia: limbic interactions with serotonin and norepinephrine. Psychopharmacology 112:S16–S34, 1993

Juorio AV: Interactions between nutritional states and some brain biogenic amines. Current Topics in Nutrition and Disease, Basic and Clinical Aspects of Nutrition and Brain Development 16:305–313, 1987

Kahn RS, Davis KL: New developments in dopamine and schizophrenia, in Psychopharmacology: The Fourth Generation of Progress. Edited by Bloom FE, Kupfer DJ. New York, Raven, 1995, pp 1193–1203

Katz HB, Davies CA, Dobbing J: Effects of undernutrition at different ages early in life and later environmental complexity on parameters of the cerebrum and hippocampus in rats. J Nutr 112:1362–1368, 1982

Keller EA, Munaro NI, Orsingher OA: Perinatal undernutrition reduces alpha and beta adrenergic receptor binding in adult rat brain. Science 215:1269–1270, 1982

Kitajima I, Yamamoto T, Ohno M, et al: Working and reference memory in rats in the three-panel runway task following dorsal hippocampal lesions. Jpn J Pharmacol 58:175–183, 1992

Klugewicz DA, Butler PD, Ciplet D, et al: Behavioral effects of prenatal protein deprivation in preweanling and adult rats. Society for Neuroscience Abstracts 21:2016, 1995

Kohsaka S, Takamatsu K, Tsukada Y: Effect of food restriction on serotonin metabolism in rat brain. Neurochem Res 5:69–79, 1980

Kovelman JA, Scheibel AB: A neurohistological correlate of schizophrenia. Biol Psychiatry 19:1601–1621, 1984

Lauder JM: Neurotransmitters as growth regulatory signals: role of receptors and second messengers. Trends Neurosci 16:233–240, 1993

Lauder JM, Bloom FE: Ontogeny of monoamine neurons in the locus coeruleus, raphe nuclei and substantia nigra of the rat. J Comp Neurol 155:469–482, 1974

Lauder JM, Krebs H: Humoral influences on brain development, in Advances in Cellular Neurobiology. New York, Academic Press, 1984, pp 3–51

Lewis PD, Patel AJ, Balazs R: Effect of undernutrition on cell generation in the adult rat brain. Brain Res 138:511–519, 1977

Lewis PD, Patel AJ, Balazs R: Effects of undernutrition on cell generation in the rat hippocampus. Brain Res 168:186–189, 1979

Liddle PF, Friston KJ, Frith CD, et al: Patterns of cerebral blood flow in schizophrenia. Br J Psychiatry 160:179–186, 1992

Lidov HGW, Molliver ME: Neocortical development after prenatal lesions of noradrenergic projections. Society for Neuroscience Abstracts 5:341, 1979

Lipska BK, Weinberger DR: Delayed effects of neonatal hippocampal damage on haloperidol-induced catalepsy and apomorphine-induced stereotypic behaviors in the rat. Developmental Brain Research 75: 213–222, 1993

Lipska BK, Jaskiw GE, Weinberger DR: Postpubertal emergence of hyperresponsiveness to stress and to amphetamine after neonatal excitotoxic hippocampal damage: a potential animal model of schizophrenia. Neuropsychopharmacology 9:67–775, 1993

Marichich ES, Molina VA, Orsingher OA: Persistent change in central catecholaminergic system after recovery of perinatally undernourished rats. J Nutr 109:1045–1050, 1979

McLardy T: Hippocampal zinc and structural deficit in brains from chronic alcoholics and some schizophrenics. Journal of Orthomolecular Psychiatry 4:32–36, 1974

Meltzer HY: Clinical studies on the mechanism of action of clozapine: the dopamine-serotonin hypothesis of schizophrenia. Psychopharmacology 99 (suppl):S18–S27, 1989

Meltzer HY: The role of serotonin in schizophrenia and the place of serotonin-dopamine antagonist antipsychotics. J Clin Psychopharmacol 15 (suppl):2S–3S, 1995

Miller M, Resnick O: Tryptophan availability: the importance of prepartum and postpartum dietary protein on brain indoleamine metabolism in rats. Exp Neurol 67:298–314, 1980

Miller M, Leahy JP, Stern WC, et al: Tryptophan availability: relation to elevated brain serotonin in developmentally protein-malnourished rats. Exp Neurol 57:142–157, 1977

Morgane PJ, Austin-LaFrance R, Bronzino J, et al: Prenatal malnutrition and development of the brain. Neurosci Biobehav Rev 17:91–128, 1993

Murray RM, Lewis SW: Is schizophrenia a neurodevelopmental disorder? BMJ 295:681–682, 1987

Musalek M, Podreka I, Walter H, et al: Regional brain function in hallucinations: a study of regional cerebral blood flow with 99m-Tc-HMPAO-SPECT in patients with auditory hallucinations, tactile hallucinations, and normal controls. Compr Psychiatry 30:99–108, 1989

Olson L, Seiger A: Early prenatal ontogeny of central monoamine neurons in the rat: fluorescence histochemical observations. Zeitschrift fur Anatomie und Entwicklungsgeschichte 137:301–316, 1972

Olton DS, Samuelson RJ: Remembrance of places passed: spatial memory in rats. J Exp Psychol Anim Behav Process 2:97–116, 1976

Olton DS, Becker JT, Handelmann GE: Hippocampus, space and memory. Behav Brain Sci 2:315–365, 1979

Pasamanick B, Rogers ME, Lilienfeld AM: Pregnancy experience and the development of behavior disorder in children. Am J Psychiatry 112:613–618, 1956

Ramanamurthy PSV: Maternal and early postnatal malnutrition and transmitter amines in rat brain. J Neurochem 28:253–254, 1977

Randt CT, Derby BM: Behavioral and brain correlations in early life nutritional deprivation. Arch Neurol 28:167–172, 1973

Resnick O, Morgane PJ: Ontogeny of the levels of serotonin in various parts of the brain in severely protein malnourished rats. Brain Res 303:163–170, 1984

Roth BL, Meltzer HY: The role of serotonin in schizophrenia, in Psychopharmacology: The Fourth Generation of Progress. Edited by Bloom FE, Kupfer DJ. New York, Raven, 1995, pp 1215–1227

Seidler FJ, Bell JM, Slotkin TA: Undernutrition and overnutrition in the neonatal rat: long-term effects on noradrenergic pathways in brain regions. Pediatr Res 27:191–197, 1990

Shoemaker WJ, Wurtman RJ: Perinatal undernutrition: accumulation of catecholamines in rat brain. Science 171:1017–1019, 1971

Shoemaker WJ, Wurtman RJ: Effect of perinatal undernutrition on the metabolism of catecholamines in the rat brain. J Nutr 103:1537–1547, 1973

Slob AK, Snow CE, Natris-Mathot E: Absence of behavioral deficits following neonatal undernutrition in the rat. Dev Psychobiol 6:177–186, 1973

Smart JL, Dobbing J: Vulnerability of developing brain, VI: relative effects of foetal and early postnatal undernutrition on reflex ontogeny and development of behavior in the rat. Brain Res 33:303–314, 1971

Smart JL, Tricklebank MD, Adlard BPF, et al: Nutritionally small-for-dates rats: their subsequent growth, regional brain 5-hydroxytryptamine turnover, and behavior. Pediatr Res 10:807–811, 1976

Sobotka TJ, Cook MP, Brodie RE: Neonatal malnutrition: neurochemical, hormonal, and behavioral manifestations. Brain Res 65:443–457, 1974

Stern WC, Miller M, Forbes WB, et al: Ontogeny of the levels of biogenic amines in various parts of the brain and in peripheral tissues in normal and protein malnourished rats. Exp Neurol 49:314–326, 1975

Suddath RL, Christison GW, Torrey EF, et al: Anatomical abnormalities in the brains of monozygotic twins discordant for schizophrenia. N Engl J Med 322:789–794, 1990

Susser ES, Lin SP: Schizophrenia after prenatal exposure to the Dutch Hunger Winter of 1944–45. Arch Gen Psychiatry 49:983–988, 1992

Susser ES, Neugebauer R, Hoek HW, et al: Schizophrenia after prenatal famine: further evidence. Arch Gen Psychiatry 53:25–31, 1996

Teyler TJ, DiScenna P: The topological anatomy of the hippocampus: a clue to its function. Brain Res Bull 12:711–719, 1984

Tonkiss J, Galler JR: Prenatal protein malnutrition and working memory performance in adult rats. Behav Brain Res 40:95–107, 1990

Tonkiss J, Galler JR, Formica RN, et al: Fetal protein malnutrition impairs acquisition of a DRL task in adult rats. Physiol Behav 48:73–77, 1990

Tonkiss J, Foster GA, Galler JR: Prenatal protein malnutrition and hippocampal function: partial reinforcement extinction effect. Brain Res Bull 27:809–813, 1991a

Tonkiss J, Galler JR, Shukitt-Hale B, et al: Prenatal protein malnutrition impairs visual discrimination learning in adult rats. Psychobiology 19: 247–250, 1991b

Tonkiss J, Schulz P, Galler JR: An analysis of spatial navigation in prenatally protein malnourished rats. Physiol Behav 55:217–224, 1994

van Kammen DP, Peters JL, van Kammen WB, et al: CSF norepinephrine in schizophrenia is elevated prior to relapse after haloperidol withdrawal. Biol Psychiatry 26:176–188, 1989

Venables PH: Hippocampal function and schizophrenia: experimental psychological evidence. Ann N Y Acad Sci 658:111–127, 1992

Waddington JL: Schizophrenia: developmental neuroscience and pathobiology. Lancet 341:531–536, 1993

Warren MA, Bedi KS: Synapse-to-neuron ratios in rat cerebellar cortex following lengthy periods of undernutrition. J Anat 170:173–182, 1990

Weinberger DR: Implications of normal brain development for the pathogenesis of schizophrenia. Arch Gen Psychiatry 44:660–669, 1987

Wiggins RC, Fuller G, Enna SJ: Undernutrition and the development of brain neurotransmitter systems. Life Sci 35:2085–2094, 1984

Part IV

Prenatal Immunological Exposures

Chapter 8

Rhesus Incompatibility and Schizophrenia

J. Megginson Hollister, Ph.D., and Alan S. Brown, M.D.

I n this chapter, we discuss the potential role of rhesus (Rh) in-compatibility and Rh hemolytic disease of the newborn (Rh HDN) in the etiology of schizophrenia. As discussed elsewhere in this volume, at least a proportion of schizophrenia cases may result from a wide range of potential factors that adversely affect neurodevelopment. As Rh incompatibility and Rh HDN are associated with abnormalities of fetal brain development, they should be considered as plausible risk factors for neurodevelopmental schizophrenia.

Rhesus incompatibility is characterized by an Rh-negative mother who carries an Rh-positive fetus. This condition may lead to Rh HDN, a hemolytic reaction marked by anemia, hepatomegaly, and neuropsychiatric consequences, including behavioral, intellectual, and motor dysfunction. The neurodevelopmental perturbations resulting from Rh HDN have some intriguing parallels to clinical and neuropathological findings in individuals who develop schizophrenia. Thus, the study of Rh incompatibility in general, and of Rh HDN in particular, provides a useful model to explore hypotheses regarding the etiopathogenesis of schizophrenia.

We first review Rh incompatibility and Rh HDN and discuss the plausibility of both as risk factors for schizophrenia. We then present empirical data on a birth cohort study that suggests an association between Rh incompatibility and schizophrenia. Finally, we suggest directions for future research in this area.

Rhesus Incompatibility and Rhesus Hemolytic Disease of the Newborn

Rhesus D Antigen

In 1939, Levine and Stetson correctly identified what would later be known as the D antigen as being responsible for a severe hemolytic reaction in a woman who had delivered a stillborn baby and was subsequently transfused with her husband's blood (Levine and Stetson 1939). A year later, the term *Rhesus* was applied to the blood-group system following work by Landsteiner and Wiener showing that rabbits, when immunized with red blood cells from rhesus monkeys, produced an antibody that reacts with human red blood cells (Landsteiner and Wiener 1940). To date, research has uncovered more than 40 different antigens on the surface of human erythrocytes that belong to the Rh blood-group system, although only 5 are common (Tippett 1987).

Of the major erythrocyte surface antigens in the Rh blood group, the D antigen is the most immunogenic and, because of this, the most clinically important (Mourant et al. 1976). Individuals who are either heterozygous (Dd) or homozygous (DD) for the D antigen are considered Rh positive; those who do not possess the D antigen are considered Rh negative (dd).

The prevalence of the Rh-negative phenotype varies worldwide. Population studies of the D antigen find that the Rh-negative phenotype ranges from 0% in a Thai population of India (Singh and Phookan 1990) to 20%–40% in the Basque people of the Pyrenees (Mourant et al. 1976). The prevalence of Rh negativity among Caucasians, African Americans, and Asians in the United States is, respectively, approximately 15%, 8%, and 0%–1% (Duerbeck and Seeds 1993).

Rhesus Incompatibility and Production of Anti-D Antibody

Rh incompatibility, defined above, can originate from the conception of a child of an Rh-negative mother, who does not possess the Rh D antigen, with an Rh-positive father, who carries the Rh D antigen. Because the Rh D antigen is inherited as an autosomal recessive trait, all offspring of homozygous Rh-positive (DD) fathers and Rh-negative (dd) mothers will be Rh-positive (Dd), whereas only 50% of the offspring of heterozygous Rh-positive (Dd) fathers and Rh-negative (dd) mothers will be Rh-positive. Thus, the probability of Rh incompatibility is highest among Rh-negative women who conceive children with homozygous Rh-positive men.

In an Rh-negative mother, the production of maternal antibody against the Rh D antigen (anti-D) can result from the birth of an Rh-positive infant, the transfusion of Rh-positive blood, or, less commonly, the miscarriage or abortion of an Rh-positive fetus. When the antibody is directed against the fetus, this is known as maternal isoimmunization. Although only 1%–2% of Rh-negative women have anti-D antibody *before* the delivery of their first Rh-positive infant, this antibody occurs in 5%–10% of Rh-negative women *after* their delivery of a D-positive, ABO-compatible infant (Foerster 1993). Mollison (1983) has suggested that the overall risk of anti-D immunization is less than 50% after infusion of relatively small amounts (<30 mL) of fetal erythrocytes, such as would occur with multiple uncomplicated deliveries. Other factors that affect the chances of maternal isoimmunization include sex of the fetus, ABO incompatibility (e.g., mother is type O and offspring is type A, B, or AB), transplacental hemorrhage, and cesarean section. Male fetuses appear to more readily initiate maternal isoimmunization against the D antigen (Renkonen and Seppala 1962; Renkonen and Timonen 1967; Scott 1976). Pregnancies that are ABO incompatible and Rh incompatible are at lowered risk for maternal immunization against the Rh D antigen, probably because fetal erythrocytes are destroyed by maternal anti-A or anti-B before maternal sensitization to the D antigen occurs (Foerster 1993). Finally, massive transplacental hemorrhage and cesarean section are associated with an increased likelihood of maternal isoimmunization due to the large amount of fetal erythrocytes coming into contact with the mother.

Rhesus Hemolytic Disease of the Newborn

If an Rh-negative woman has been isoimmunized against the D antigen, she has the potential of delivering an Rh-positive child with Rh HDN. Hemolytic disease rarely affects a firstborn Rh-positive infant (see above probability of maternal isoimmunization), and the incidence/severity of HDN is known to be about fivefold greater (in terms of stillbirth rate) in second- and later-affected neonates than in first-affected neonates (Mollison 1993). Hemolytic disease results from the lysis of fetal erythrocytes by transplacentally acquired maternal erythrocyte alloantibodies (anti-D). The erythrolysis occurs initially in the fetal liver and subsequently in the spleen of the fetus and newborn, leading to excessive breakdown of hemoglobin and subsequent hyperbilirubinemia.

The clinical manifestations of HDN are varied. Outcomes include early spontaneous abortion and stillbirth in an unknown percentage of pregnancies. Among live births, hydrops fetalis, a severely edematous condition that is often fatal, develops in approximately 20%; hepatomegaly and moderate anemia occur in approximately 30%; and the remaining 50% experience mild or no anemia with spontaneous recovery (Duerbeck and Seeds 1993).

Additionally, newborns with hemolytic disease have higher rates of respiratory difficulties, such as asphyxia and pulmonary edema (Halitsky 1990). Newborns who present with hepatomegaly and moderate anemia are at risk of developing hyperbilirubinemia postpartum. If left untreated, hyperbilirubinemia can, within the first few days of life, result in kernicterus, a condition characterized by the accumulation of neurotoxic bilirubin in specific brain structures (see subsection below titled "Type and Timing of Neuropathology"). Those infants who survive kernicterus may manifest any of the following clinical sequelae: choreoathetosis, sensorineural hearing deficits, and/or mental retardation (Watchko and Oski 1992).

The prognosis for infants born with HDN began improving in the 1950s with the routine use of exchange transfusions for affected newborns. Further improvement came in 1963 with the introduction of intrauterine transfusion for affected fetuses. Fortunately, with the advent of anti-D prophylaxis in 1968 (e.g., passive immunization of Rh-negative mothers with Rh D immune globulin, or "Rhogam"), maternal isoimmunization has become less common, and the frequency of HDN has declined by between five- and tenfold (Mollison 1993).

Plausibility of Rh Incompatibility as a Risk Factor for Schizophrenia

Rh HDN and schizophrenia share several important features that support the plausibility of Rh incompatibility in the etiology of at least some cases of schizophrenia (Table 8–1). These features include 1) type and timing of neuropathology, 2) association with obstetric complications, and 3) clinical manifestations of Rh HDN survivors and individuals destined to develop schizophrenia.

Type and Timing of Neuropathology

The placental transfer of maternal anti-D in Rh HDN is under way by the second trimester (Adinolphi 1985), during which fetal expression of HDN has been demonstrated (Mollison 1993). The D alloantibodies are capable of perturbing fetal neurodevelopment through at least two different mechanisms. In the first, hemolysis results in chronic fetal hypoxia that may affect multiple brain regions; the hippocampus is one brain region particularly vulnerable to hypoxia (Ben Ari 1992; Rorke 1992). In the second, as discussed earlier, hyperbilirubinemia may result in kernicterus, leading to permanent brain damage to the basal ganglia, hippocampus, thalamus, dentate nucleus of the cerebellum, and other regions (Larroche 1984; Rorke 1992).

Abnormalities in most of these brain regions have been demonstrated in both neuroimaging and postmortem studies of schizo-

Table 8–1. Parallels between rhesus (Rh) incompatibility and schizophrenia

	Rh incompatibility/ Rh HDN	Schizophrenia
Neuropathology	Basal ganglia	Basal ganglia
	Hippocampus	Hippocampus
	Other areas	Other areas
Timing of insult	Second and third trimester (definite)	Second trimester (?)
Obstetric complications	Perinatal	Pre- and perinatal
Childhood history	Neuromotor abnormalities	Neuromotor abnormalities
	Anxiety, emotional instability	Anxiety, emotional instability
	Lowered IQ (?)	Lowered IQ (?)
Maternal immunology	Definite	Possible
Genetics	Autosomal recessive (Rh incompatibility)	Likely multifactorial
	Multifactorial (Rh HDN)	
Epidemiology	On the decline (definite)	On the decline (?)

Note. Rh HDN = Rhesus hemolytic disease of the newborn.

phrenia (Bogerts and Falkai 1991), and a second-trimester insult is proposed on the basis of neuronal migration disturbances (Akbarian et al. 1993; Kovelman and Scheibel 1984) and epidemiological findings implicating prenatal influenza in this illness (Mednick et al. 1988; O'Callaghan et al. 1991).

Obstetric Complications

As noted earlier, certain obstetric complications occur secondarily to Rh incompatibility. In particular, complications that have hypoxic and anoxic qualities are observed among hemolytic neonates. Likewise, an association between schizophrenia and increased number of obstetric complications has been reported (M. H. Jones et al. 1998; McNeil 1988). Although no specific obstetric complication has been pinpointed as a critical risk factor in schizophrenia, McNeil (1988) has proposed that the common denominator of many of the complications appears to be hypoxia. This assertion is consistent with Mednick's (1970) proposal that anoxia from obstetric complications could selectively damage the hippocampus and, in interaction with unidentified genetic factors, result in later development of mental disturbance in individuals at high risk for schizophrenia.

Clinical Manifestations in HDN Survivors and Individuals Who Subsequently Develop Schizophrenia

Certain psychological, intellectual, and neuromotor abnormalities have been observed in children who survived HDN. The majority of follow-up studies of survivors of HDN included evaluations conducted between infancy and early childhood, and a few studies followed subjects until 10–14 years of age. Psychological abnormalities included emotional instability, fearfulness, excitability, anxiety and tenseness, lack of persistence, lack of conscientiousness, and social immaturity (Gerrard 1952; Rosta et al. 1971; Stewart et al. 1970; Turner et al. 1975; W. Walker et al. 1974). Other studies of HDN survivors did not examine psychological outcomes (Ellis 1980; M. H. Jones et al. 1954; Knobbe et al. 1979; Van Praagh 1961; White et al. 1978).

HDN survivors also have higher rates of neurological abnormalities, including choreoathetosis, probably as a result of lesions in the basal ganglia due to intranatal asphyxia or postpartum hyperbilirubinemia (Bock and Winkel 1976; Ellis 1980; Richings 1973; Rosta et al. 1971; Van Praagh 1961; W. Walker et al. 1974). Moreover, studies have reported intellectual abnormalities, including lower-than-average IQ (Rosta et al. 1971; Turner et al. 1975), difficulty in acquiring new vocabulary or in learning language (Phibbs et al. 1971; W. Walker et al. 1974), and deficient visual-perceptual-motor organization (Stewart et al. 1970).

These investigations have many limitations. Most of the studies included only those individuals who underwent intrauterine and exchange transfusions (for treatment of HDN); hence, the subjects are probably not representative of all individuals affected by HDN. In addition, many of the studies used small sample sizes, weak or vague methodology, and questionable or no controls. Finally, no follow-up studies of HDN into adulthood were located, a fact that may explain the lack of associations between HDN and psychosis.

Nonetheless, the findings reported bear some similarities to psychosocial, intellectual, and neuromotor abnormalities observed in children and adolescents destined to develop schizophrenia (see Table 8–1). Emotional instability (Janes et al. 1983; John et al. 1982; Olin et al. 1955; Schwartzman et al. 1985; Watt 1972, 1978; Watt and Lubensky 1976; Watt et al. 1982), poor affective control (Parnas and Jorgensen 1989; Parnas et al. 1982), social anxiety, withdrawal, aloofness, disruptiveness (P. Jones et al. 1995), less motivation, and more verbal negativity (Janes et al. 1983; Watt et al. 1982) have all been reported both in children at high risk for schizophrenia and in those who later developed the illness. Impaired intellectual functioning has been described both before development of the illness and after its onset (Fenton et al. 1994; P. Jones et al. 1995). Choreoathetosis and other neuromotor disturbances, including poor motor skills and abnormal hand posture, have been observed in infants and children who developed schizophrenia in adulthood (Mednick and Silverton 1988; E. F. Walker et al. 1994). These abnormalities have been linked to structural impairment of the basal ganglia (E. F. Walker 1994), a brain region affected by HDN (see above).

Evidence Supporting Rh Incompatibility as a Risk Factor for Schizophrenia

With this in mind, we undertook a study, using the Danish Perinatal Cohort, to examine whether Rh incompatibility is a risk factor for schizophrenia (Hollister et al. 1996). A further, more personal, reason for pursuing this question was that the first author's sister, who has suffered from schizophrenia for many years, is Rh incompatible with her mother, and jaundice was noted at birth.

Study Design

The Danish Perinatal Cohort consists of 9,182 infants born to 9,006 women between 1959 and 1961 at University Hospital in Copenhagen, Denmark. Serological data were recorded for more than one-third of the offspring in the sample and for the majority of the mothers. Nearly 40% of the offspring with blood data were from Rh-negative women, a far higher percentage than that observed in the general Danish population (17%). This indicated that blood sampling was selectively biased to pregnancies that warranted serological examination for reasons such as risk of Rh incompatibility or prematurity.

Because a relatively small number of female cohort members developed schizophrenia, only males were included in the study. Subjects were separated into two groups according to whether or not they were Rh incompatible with their mothers, as assessed through retrospective examination of mother and offspring blood types. An Rh-incompatible group of 535 men and an Rh-compatible group of 1,332 men were ascertained. In 1992–1993, data on schizophrenia diagnosis for cohort members were obtained through a search of the Danish Psychiatric Hospital Register. The Danish Psychiatric Hospital Register includes data on all psychiatric hospitalizations of the entire Danish population. These data include diagnoses, dates of hospitalization(s), and age at hospitalization(s).

Study Findings

We found that 11 individuals in the Rh-incompatible group (2.1%) and 10 individuals in the Rh-compatible group (0.8%) had developed schizophrenia by 1993 (relative risk [RR] = 2.78, 95% confidence interval [CI] = 1.2–6.6). The fact that Rh HDN rarely affects firstborn Rh-incompatible subjects provided us with the opportunity to refine our hypothesis; higher rates of schizophrenia would be found in nonfirstborn subjects. We therefore separated the subjects by birth order and compared the rate of schizophrenia in firstborn individuals with the rate in second- and later-born individuals. As hypothesized, the rate of schizophrenia was not significantly different in firstborn Rh-incompatible and Rh-compatible individuals (1.1% vs. 0.7%); however, among second- and later-born individuals, the rate of schizophrenia was significantly greater in the Rh-incompatible than in the Rh-compatible group (2.6% vs. 0.8%, respectively; RR = 3.32, 95% CI = 1.0–10.6) (Hollister et al. 1996).

The limitations of the study included the relatively small sample size, which could have increased the likelihood of a chance finding, and the lack of a female sample. The small number of females with a diagnosis of schizophrenia in our sample precluded a meaningful analysis of the data. We attributed the lack of females to their later age at schizophrenia onset. Despite these limitations, we believe Rh incompatibility to be a compelling risk factor for schizophrenia, as this hypothesis is concordant with growing evidence that genetic and immunological factors play important roles in schizophrenia. We shall therefore discuss the genetics and immunology of Rh incompatibility in the context of our current understanding of these putative causes of schizophrenia.

Genetics

A wealth of evidence has implicated genetic factors in the etiology of schizophrenia, although in most cases the inheritance pattern appears to be explained only by invoking complex genetic models such as epistatic and gene–environment interactions (see Chapter 2, this volume). Unlike other proposed risk factors for schizophrenia, Rh incompatibility is clearly a genetic disorder. Yet although the inheritance pattern of the Rh D antigen follows simple Mendelian laws (i.e., autosomal recessive), Rh HDN does not appear to be inherited in this manner. Indeed, in the vast majority of cases of Rh incompatibility in second or later births (prior to the institution of prophylaxis), the infant was not affected. Although the reasons for the development of anti-D antibodies and the occurrence of Rh HDN are poorly understood, we shall provide some examples (see section below titled "Directions for Future Research").

Immunology

Emerging data point to a possible autoimmune etiology in schizophrenia (see Chapter 9, this volume). It is therefore of particular interest that Rh HDN exemplifies an illness with neurological consequences that is secondary to adverse prenatal effects of a maternal antibody. Hence, if our findings are replicated, Rh HDN may serve as a model to validate immunological hypotheses of schizophrenia and elucidate autoimmune pathogenic mechanisms in this disorder.

Directions for Future Research

Our future efforts in investigating an association between Rh incompatibility and risk for schizophrenia will focus on four major areas: replication studies, genetic and environmental interactions, epidemiological studies, and exploration of related phenomena.

Replication Studies

We are currently initiating a study to replicate our finding of an association between Rh incompatibility and risk for schizophrenia, using a much larger cohort in Helsinki, Finland, born between 1959 and 1969. Our group will compare the risk of schizophrenia in the offspring of 2,000 Rh-incompatible pregnancies at high risk for HDN and 4,000 Rh-compatible pregnancies. In addition to the larger sample size, other advantages offered by use of this cohort include comprehensive data on prenatal and perinatal variables related to Rh HDN (e.g., maternal antibody titers, hemoglobin and bilirubin values, number of exchange transfusions, obstetric complications), inclusion of female subjects, and the opportunity to locate subjects and first-degree relatives at a later date for further study. The larger sample size should enable us to better examine whether any clinical or demographic differences exist between the two groups and should allow for analysis of HDN severity and risk for schizophrenia.

Genetic and Environmental Interactions

Epistatic and gene–environment interactions might predispose a pregnancy to Rh HDN. ABO incompatibility (e.g., mother is type O and offspring is type A, B, or AB), which is also genetically determined, decreases the risk for maternal immunization against the Rh D antigen via the destruction of fetal red blood cells by the naturally occurring anti-A or anti-B antibodies in the maternal circulation before Rh sensitization takes place (Foerster 1993). Therefore, future studies of Rh incompatibility and schizophrenia should also examine ABO status. These studies have the potential to illuminate a possible epistatic interaction in schizophrenia.

A gene–environment interaction would be exemplified by massive transplacental hemorrhage or cesarean section, which would increase the likelihood of isoimmunization in Rh-incompatible pregnancies. Thus, Rh HDN (the phenotype) may only be expressed in the presence of specific environmental factors. Intriguingly, many investigators have proposed the same type of model for schizophrenia. These factors will be investigated using extensive data on perinatal complications from our planned replication study.

Epidemiological Studies

Concordance between variations in place and time of two disorders provides important clues that they may share a common etiology. For Rh HDN, morbidity and mortality have been significantly reduced since the introduction of exchange and intrauterine transfusions in the late 1940s and early 1960s, respectively, and the introduction of Rhogam for Rh-incompatible pregnancies in 1968–1970 (Mollison 1993). The annual rates of Rh HDN in the United States declined from 45.1 to 20.6 per 10,000 total births (live and still) between 1970 and 1975 (Wysowski et al. 1979), plateauing at around 10–15 births per 10,000 annually since 1979 (Chavez et al. 1991).

If Rh incompatibility, via Rh HDN, is important in the etiology of schizophrenia, one might predict a decline in schizophrenia approximately two decades after the incidence of HDN had been significantly reduced. Thus, the effects of this decline on the rate of schizophrenia would probably not be noticeable for at least several more years, unless the use of exchange and intrauterine transfusions dramatically reduced neurodevelopmental abnormalities leading to schizophrenia. On the other hand, it is also possible that improved prenatal and neonatal care, by improving survival rates of erythroblastotic fetuses and neonates, may cause a paradoxical increase in schizophrenia due to those compromised offspring surviving the neonatal period. Thus, any ameliorating effect of anti-D prophylaxis (Rh HDN prevention) on rates of schizophrenia may be canceled out by an increase in schizophrenia among those fetuses and newborns who continue to develop HDN but who have improved chances of survival because of advancing medical technology.

As discussed earlier, population studies demonstrate marked variation in the prevalence of Rh negativity in different regions, ethnic groups, and time periods. Thus, comparisons of the geographic, ethnic, and temporal distributions of Rh negativity and schizophrenia could also prove valuable.

Finally, epidemiological studies suggest that increased maternal age might represent a risk factor for schizophrenia in offspring (Hare and Moran 1979). This finding might be explained by the fact that nonfirstborn Rh-incompatible children are at increased risk of HDN.

Exploration of Related Phenomena

ABO incompatibility, like Rh incompatibility, may cause jaundice, a symptom that occurs in about incompatible pregnancies. This suggests that ABO incompatibility should also be investigated as a potential risk factor for schizophrenia.

Conclusion

Rh HDN is a condition that affects early brain development, that possesses both genetic and immunological determinants, and, as such, that could account for a collection of compelling, yet often disparate, findings in schizophrenia. We have found suggestive preliminary evidence from a birth cohort study that Rh incompatibility is a risk factor for schizophrenia. Although future attempts at replication are warranted, this line of investigation holds promise for identifying a preventable cause of schizophrenia, a possibility that only recently seemed far out of reach.

References

Adinolphi M: The development of the human blood–CSF–brain barrier. Dev Med Child Neurol 27:532–537, 1985

Akbarian S, Vinuela A, Kim JJ, et al: Distorted distribution of nicotinamide-adenine dinucleotide phosphate-diaphorase neurons in temporal lobe of schizophrenics implies anomalous cortical development. Arch Gen Psychiatry 50:178–187, 1993

Ben Ari Y: Effect of anoxia and aglycemia on the adult and immature hippocampus. Biol Neonate 62:225–230, 1992

Bock JE, Winkel S: A follow-up study on infants who received intra-uterine transfusions because of severe rhesus haemolytic disease. Acta Obstet Gynecol Scand Suppl 53:37–40, 1976

Bogerts B, Falkai P: Clinical and neurodevelopmental aspects of brain pathology in schizophrenia, in Developmental Neuropathology of Schizophrenia. Edited by Mednick SA, Cannon TD, Barr CE, et al. New York, Plenum, 1991, pp 93–120

Chavez GF, Mulinare J, Edmonds LD: Epidemiology of Rh hemolytic disease of the newborn in the United States. JAMA 265:3270–3274, 1991

Duerbeck NB, Seeds JW: Rhesus immunization in pregnancy: a review. Obstet Gynecol Surv 48:801–810, 1993

Ellis MI: Follow-up study of survivors after intra-uterine transfusion. Dev Med Child Neurol 22:48–54, 1980

Fenton WS, Wyatt RJ, McGlashan TH: Risk factors for spontaneous dyskinesia in schizophrenia. Arch Gen Psychiatry 51:643–650, 1994

Foerster J: Alloimmune hemolytic anemias, in Wintrobe's Clinical Hematology, 9th Edition. Edited by Lee GR, Birthell TC, Foerster J, et al. Philadelphia, PA, Lea & Febiger, 1993, pp 1146–1169

Gerrard J: Kernicterus. Brain 75:527–571, 1952

Halitsky V: Sequelae in children who survived in utero fetal transfusion: a comparison with those who underwent postpartum exchange transfusion, in Obstetrical Events and Developmental Sequelae. Edited by Tegami N. Boca Raton, FL, CRC, 1990, pp 111–126

Hare EH, Moran PAP: Raised parental age in psychiatric patients: evidence for the constitutional hypothesis. Br J Psychiatry 134:169–177, 1979

Hollister JM, Laing P, Mednick SA: Rhesus incompatibility as a risk factor for schizophrenia in male adults. Arch Gen Psychiatry 53:19–24, 1996

Janes CL, Weeks DG, Worland J: School behavior in adolescent children of parents with mental disorder. J Nerv Ment Dis 171:234–240, 1983

John RS, Mednick SA, Schulsinger F: Teacher reports as a predictor of schizophrenia and borderline schizophrenia: a Bayesian decision analysis. J Abnorm Psychol 91:399–413, 1982

Jones MH, Sauds R, Hyman CB, et al: Longitudinal study of the incidence of central nervous system damage following erythroblastosis fetalis. Pediatr 14:346–350, 1954

Jones P, Murray R, Rodgers B: Childhood risk factors for adult schizophrenia in a general birth cohort at age 43 years, in Neural Development in Schizophrenia: Theory and Research. Edited by Mednick SA, Hollister JM. New York, Plenum, 1995, pp 151–176

Jones PB, Rantakallio P, Hartikainen AL, et al: Schizophrenia as a long-term outcome of pregnancy, delivery, and perinatal complications: a 28-year follow-up of the 1966 north Finland general population birth cohort. Am J Psychiatry 155:355–364, 1998,1,8

Knobbe T, Meier P, Wenar C, et al:Psychological development of children who received intrauterine transfusions. Am J Obstet Gynecol 133: 877–879, 1979

Kovelman JA, Scheibel AB: A neurohistological correlate of schizophrenia. Biol Psychiatry 19:1601–1621, 1984

Landsteiner K, Wiener AS: An agglutinable factor in human blood recognized by immune sera for rhesus blood (letter). Proc Soc Exp Biol Med 43:223, 1940

Larroche JC: Perinatal brain damage, in Greenfield's Neuropathology. Edited by Adams JH, Corsellis JAN, Duchen LW. New York, John Wiley & Sons, 1984, pp 458–480

Levine P, Stetson RE: An unusual case of intra-group agglutination. JAMA 113:126–127, 1939

McNeil TF: Obstetric factors and perinatal injuries, in Handbook of Schizophrenia. Edited by Tsuang MT, Simpson JC. Amsterdam, Elsevier, 1988, pp 319–344

Mednick SA: Breakdown in individuals at high risk for schizophrenia: possible predispositional perinatal factors. Mental Hygiene 54:50–61, 1970

Mednick SA, Silverton L: High-risk studies of the etiology of schizophrenia, in Handbook of Schizophrenia, Vol 3: Nosology, Epidemiology, and Genetics. Edited by Tsuang M. Amsterdam, Elsevier Science, 1988, pp 543–562

Mednick SA, Machon RA, Huttunen MO, et al: Adult schizophrenia following prenatal exposure to an influenza epidemic. Arch Gen Psychiatry 45:189–192, 1988

Mollison PL: Blood Transfusion in Clinical Medicine, 7th Edition. Oxford, England, Blackwell Scientific, 1983

Mollison PL: Haemolytic disease of the fetus and newborn, in Blood Transfusion in Clinical Medicine. Edited by Mollison PL, Engelfriet CP, Contreras M. Oxford, England, Blackwell Scientific, 1993, pp 543–591

Mourant AE, Kopec AC, Domaniewska-Sobczak K: The Rhesus blood groups, in The Distribution of the Human Blood Groups and Other Biochemical Polymorphisms. Edited by Mourant AE, Kopec AC, Domaniewska-Sobczak K. Oxford, England, Oxford University Press, 1976, pp 11–13

O'Callaghan E, Sham PC, Takei N, et al: Schizophrenia after prenatal exposure to 1957 A2 influenza epidemic. Lancet 337:1248–1250, 1991

Olin SS, John RS, Mednick SA: Assessing the predictive value of teacher reports in a high risk sample for schizophrenia: an ROC analysis. Schizophr Res 16:53–66, 1995

Parnas J, Jorgensen A: Premorbid psychopathology in schizophrenia spectrum. Br J Psychiatry 155:623–627, 1989

Parnas J, Schulsinger F, Schulsinger H, et al: Behavioral precursors of schizophrenia spectrum: a prospective study. Arch Gen Psychiatry 47:1023–1028, 1982

Phibbs RH, Harvin D, Jones G, et al: Development of children who had received intra-uterine transfusions. Pediatrics 47:689–697, 1971

Renkonen KO, Seppala M: The sex of the sensitizing Rh-positive child. Annales Medicinae Experimentalis et Biologiae Fenniae 40:108–110, 1962

Renkonen KO, Timonen S: Factors influencing the immunization of Rh-negative mothers. J Med Genet 4:166–168, 1967

Richings J: Later progress of infants who received transfusions in utero for severe rhesus hemolytic disease. Lancet 1220–1223, 1973

Rorke LB: Perinatal brain damage, in Greenfield's Neuropathology, 5th Edition. Edited by Adams JH, Duchen LW. New York, Oxford University Press, 1992, pp 639–708

Rosta J, Makoi Z, Bekefi D, et al: Neonatal pathologic jaundice: seven to nine years follow-up. Acta Paediatrica Academiae Scientiarum Hungaricae 12:317–321, 1971

Schwartzman AE, Ledingham JE, Serbin LA: Identification of children at risk for adult schizophrenia: a longitudinal study. International review of Applied Psychology 34:363–380, 1985

Scott JR: Immunologic risks to fetuses from maternal to fetal transfer of erythrocytes. Proceedings of the Symposium on Rh Antibody–Mediated Immunosuppression, Raritan, NJ, Ortho Research Institute, 1976

Singh TS, Phookan MN: A note on the frequency of ABO and rhesus blood groups in four Thai populations of Assam (India) and their position among Mongoloids of this region. Anthropologischer Anzeiger 48:29–35, 1990

Stewart RR, Walker W, Savage RD: A developmental study of cognitive and personality characteristics associated with haemolytic disease of the newborn. Dev Med Child Neurol 12:16–26, 1970

Tippett P: Rh blood group system: the D antigen and high- and low-frequency Rh antigens, in Blood Group Systems. Edited by Vengelen-Tyler V, Pierce SR. Arlington, VA, American Association of Blood Banks, 1987, pp 120–155

Turner JH, Hutchinson DL, Hayashi TT, et al: Fetal and maternal risks associated with intrauterine transfusion procedures. Am J Obstet Gynecol 123:251–256, 1975

Van Praagh R: Diagnosis of kernicterus in the neonatal period. Pediatrics 27:870–876, 1961

Walker EF: Developmentally moderated expressions of the neuropathology underlying schizophrenia. Schizophr Bull 20:453–480, 1994

Walker EF, Savoie T, Davis D: Neuromotor precursors of schizophrenia. Schizophr Bull 20:441–451, 1994

Walker W, Ellis MI, Ellis E, et al: A follow-up study of survivors of Rh-haemolytic disease. Dev Med Child Neurol 16:592–611, 1974

Watchko JF, Oski FA: Kernicterus in preterm newborns: past, present, and future. Pediatrics 90:707–715, 1992

Watt NF: Longitudinal changes in the social behavior of children hospitalized for schizophrenia as adults. J Nerv Ment Dis 155:42–54, 1972

Watt NF: Patterns of childhood social development in adult schizophrenics. Arch Gen Psychiatry 35:160–165, 1978

Watt NF, Lubensky AW: Childhood roots of schizophrenia. J Consult Clin Psychol 44:363–375, 1976

Watt NF, Grubb TW, Erlenmeyer-Kimling L: Social, emotional and intellectual behavior at school among children at high risk for schizophrenia. J Consult Clin Psychol 50:171–181, 1982

White CA, Goplerud CP, Kisker CT, et al: Intrauterine fetal transfusion, 1965–1976, with an assessment of the surviving children. Am J Obstet Gynecol 130:933–940, 1978

Wysowski DK, Flynt JW, Goldberg MF, et al: Rh hemolytic disease: epidemiologic surveillance in the United States 1968–1975. JAMA 242: 1376–1379, 1979

Chapter 9

Heat Shock Proteins and Autoimmune Mechanisms of Disease in Schizophrenia

David H. Strauss, M.D.

Immune and autoimmune mechanisms have been implicated in many disease states, including those that affect the central nervous system (CNS). A convergence of evidence from clinic and laboratory has lent support to a theory that abnormal immune mechanisms may play a role in the etiology or pathophysiology of schizophrenia. The findings presented in Chapter 8 suggest that an abnormal prenatal immune response—the production of Rhesus D antigen (RhD) antibody directed against fetal tissues—could increase liability to schizophrenia. In this chapter I provide further evidence supporting a link between schizophrenia and autoimmune pathology. The central question to be considered here is whether the autoimmune abnormalities observed in schizophrenia represent evidence of pathological immune mechanisms related to the cause or course of the disorder or constitute only indirectly or secondarily related phenomena.

While not necessarily confined to the prenatal period, the findings to be presented may shed further light on—and be informed by—material described in the other chapters of this book. For instance, as proposed by Wright and colleagues in Chapter 4, one plausible mechanism by which prenatal infection might lead to schizophrenia is through induction of autoantibodies that attack

215

the fetal brain; and, given the important role of genes in the immune response, this scenario can be better understood using the gene–environment interaction models described by Malaspina et al. in Chapter 2. Therefore, I have devoted considerable discussion to several causal pathways that link autoimmunity with genetic diathesis and infectious exposures in the etiopathogenesis of schizophrenia.

Characteristics of Classical Autoimmune Diseases Relevant to Schizophrenia

Autoimmune disorders, including multiple sclerosis, insulin-dependent diabetes mellitus (IDDM), and rheumatoid arthritis are common clinical disorders (Sinha et al. 1990). Clinical similarities between many of the autoimmune illnesses and schizophrenia, such as those related to onset, course, and gender effects, are interesting and often cited. Epidemiological evidence demonstrating a negative association between schizophrenia and rheumatoid arthritis has been used to support a theory of shared genetic vulnerability. For example, Knight (1985) has speculated that schizophrenia and rheumatoid arthritis are coded for by mutually exclusive alleles of the same gene. In IDDM, both negative and positive associations with schizophrenia have been reported (see Chapter 4, this volume). Other characteristics of autoimmune diseases relevant to an autoimmune theory of schizophrenia emerge from a review of etiological considerations, pathophysiological processes, and models of human autoimmune disease.

Etiological Considerations: Genetic Diathesis/Environmental Trigger

Genetic factors are believed to influence development of both autoimmune diseases and schizophrenia. In autoimmune disease, as in schizophrenia, the interaction of multiple genes is presumed.

Gene–environment interactions are of importance in both autoimmune disease and schizophrenia, and the partial concordance rates for monozygotic twins with schizophrenia (30%–50% concordance), IDDM (30%), and multiple sclerosis (5%–30%) supports this notion. The association of many autoimmune diseases with prior infection suggests that the critical environmental influence in autoimmune disease may be a virus or other environmental pathogen (Table 9–1). This is an idea consistent with some recently proposed etiological models for schizophrenia, such as that of Wright and Murray (1993) and Wright and colleagues (see Chapter 4, this volume). Wright et al. have proposed that autoimmune mechanisms might explain observed epidemiological associations of schizophrenia with influenza infection. Evidence of viral exposure (Crow 1983) and epidemiological evidence that in utero exposure to influenza increases the risk for subsequent development of schizophrenia (Mednick et al. 1988) are consistent with an infectious basis for schizophrenia. Recent studies reporting linkage of schizophrenia with a gene on chromosome 6, a site that may lie within the major histocompatibility locus, provide a further, albeit indirect, association among schizophrenia, genes, and immunity (Wang et al. 1995). Finally, our data on serum autoantibodies to the 60-kilodalton (kD) heat shock protein (hsp60) in patients with schizophrenia also link schizophrenia, infection, and autoimmunity; these findings are presented later in this chapter.

Table 9–1. Autoimmune diseases linked to infectious agents via molecular mimicry

Disease	Putative infectious agent
Rheumatic heart disease	Group A streptococcus
Rheumatoid arthritis	Mycobacterium tuberculosis
Sydenham's chorea	Group A streptococcus
Multiple sclerosis	Ebstein-Barr virus, hepatitis B virus
Schizophrenia	?

Pathophysiological Processes: Mechanisms of CNS Autoimmune Disease Relevant to Schizophrenia

Noninflammatory Mechanisms

The absence of gliosis and other hallmarks of old or active inflammation is a consistent finding in postmortem studies in schizophrenia and has been used to refute theories of immune pathogenesis. However, autoantibodies are known to exert diverse effects on cells and tissues and can cause CNS disease by binding to functionally important cellular components, inducing dysfunction without creating inflammatory damage or gross pathological change. Furthermore, the vast repertoire of cytokine messengers involved in the immune response is known to influence neural functions, including those related to growth, development, and synaptic transmission. These cytokines may play an important mediating role in the pathophysiology of CNS disease, including schizophrenia (Strauss and Printz 1996).

In autoimmune processes, autoantibodies can mimic natural ligands, inducing allosteric changes in receptors and interacting with cell surface and intracytoplasmic components (see Table 9–1). For example, in Graves' disease, autoantibodies bind to the thyroid-stimulating hormone (TSH) receptor, activate the thyroid, and produce clinical hyperthyroidism (Smith et al. 1988). Myasthenia gravis is a neuromuscular disorder characterized by progressive weakness and fatigability. Although autoantibodies in myasthenia gravis trigger destruction of the postsynaptic membrane through an inflammatory mechanism, a number of autoantibodies with acetylcholine receptor antagonist properties have been identified (Richman et al. 1990). In Lambert-Eaton syndrome, a related disease of the neuromuscular junction, autoantibodies target the presynaptic voltage-gated calcium channel, decreasing acetylcholine release and neuromuscular junction transmission (Newsome-Davis 1988). In stiff-man syndrome, a disorder characterized by muscular rigidity and painful muscular spasms, impaired transmission at gamma-aminobutyric acid (GABA) synapses has been linked to the presence of autoantibodies to glutamic acid decarboxylase (GAD), the enzyme that catalyzes the rate-limiting step in GABA synthesis (Solimena et al. 1990). An as yet incompletely characterized autoantibody–antigen reaction has been specifically associated with psychosis in patients with neuropsychiatric lupus erythematosus. Serum levels of these antineuronal antibodies were found to correlate with severity of psychosis in a small series of cases (Bonfa et al. 1987). A final example is paraneoplastic degenerative syndrome, in which antiglutamate subunit antibodies have been found to increase receptor sensitivity to glutamate and hasten the neuronal degeneration typical of the disease (Gahring et al. 1995). Knight (1985) theorized that schizophrenia may result from antibody-mediated dysregulation of dopaminergic transmission, although there is no direct empirical support for this theory to date.

Loss of Self-Tolerance in the Nervous System

Under normal circumstances, the immune system differentiates the body's own proteins and cells from foreign ones through an incompletely understood mechanism referred to as *tolerance.* When this process fails and a loss of self-tolerance occurs, the immune system may target and attack the body's own tissues as if they were foreign, causing autoimmune disease. The immune system's arsenal is large and varied; a cascade of cellular, antibody, and cytokine responses are mobilized for surveillance, identification, and elimination of foreign organisms. Each of these elements of the immune response contributes to pathogenesis in autoimmune disease.

Environmental stressors, such as exposure to infectious agents, toxins, or trauma, are believed to trigger the breakdown in self-tolerance that leads to autoimmunity. One explanatory model for autoantibody production is termed "molecular mimicry," a process that depends on the presence of a structural similarity between a foreign protein, which initiates an immune response, and a self-protein (Cohen 1990). Antibodies raised against the foreign protein (e.g., a viral antigen) will also recognize the self-protein and will therefore trigger an autoimmune reaction. In an alternative model, autoantibodies following infection result from a physical association of cellular proteins with viral proteins—for example, through the incorporation of cellular proteins into viral particles (Zinker-nagel et al. 1990). When the incorporated cellular protein is presented to the immune system in conjunction with the viral antigens, an immune response to the self-antigen can be triggered, with subsequent loss of tolerance to that antigen. Finally, blood–brain barrier disruption, with exposure of previously sequestered antigenic determinants, can promote immune-mediated pathology. Toxins, infection, and trauma have each been associated with etiopathogenesis in schizophrenia. That these factors may exert their influence in schizophrenia by triggering the breakdown in self-tolerance that underlies autoimmunity is an intriguing possibility.

Sydenham's Chorea and Rasmussen's Encephalitis as Models for Schizophrenia

Sydenham's chorea and Rasmussen's encephalitis are diseases of the CNS in which autoimmunity triggered by environmental factors gives rise to neuropsychiatric syndromes via effects on neural transmission. Although the comparison may be limited, in that both Sydenham's and Rasmussen's involve inflammatory changes not seen in schizophrenia, these disease models contribute elements useful to the development of a model of autoimmunity in schizophrenia.

Sydenham's Chorea

Sydenham's chorea provides an example of a neuropsychiatric disease putatively linked to a cross-reacting antibody triggered by an infectious agent (Figure 9–1). Sydenham's represents a classical manifestation of rheumatic fever, a potential sequelae of Group A

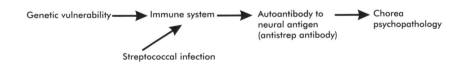

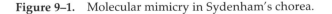

Figure 9–1.   Molecular mimicry in Sydenham's chorea.

streptococcal infection. Patients with the disorder develop adventitious choreic movements, other motor disturbances, and psychiatric symptoms. Sydenham's chorea usually occurs in childhood or early adolescence and has a female predominance. It also occurs at an increased rate in family members of affected patients.

Significant psychopathology has been described in patients with Sydenham's chorea, many of whom manifest overt obsessive-compulsive symptoms (Swedo et al. 1993). In a retrospective chart review of 969 hospitalized psychiatric patients, Wilcox and Nasrallah (1986) found that psychotic patients were more likely than nonpsychotic patients to have a history of rheumatic chorea. In a prospective study of 29 individuals with Sydenham's chorea and matched surgical control subjects, the same investigators demonstrated that patients with chorea were more likely to have psychiatric symptoms at 10-year follow-up (Wilcox and Nasrallah 1988).

Chorea in Sydenham's has been linked to central presynaptic dopaminergic dysfunction and other dopaminergic changes (Naidu and Narasimhachari 1980; Nausieda et al. 1983). In addition, pathological changes in the basal ganglia have been recognized in postmortem studies. Husby and colleagues (1976) demonstrated antibodies against a cytoplasmic structure in caudate and subthalamic neurons in 47% of patients with Sydenham's chorea. Autoantibody titers correlated with disease severity. Although no specific CNS antigen has been identified to date, Kiessling and co-workers (1993) have suggested that antibodies bind to the D_2 dopamine receptor.

These findings may be relevant to neural dysfunction in schizophrenia. It is noteworthy that choreiform movements have been demonstrated in schizophrenia in the absence of medication effects, structural abnormalities are widely cited, and dopaminergic receptor changes are reported (Wong et al. 1986).

Rasmussen's Encephalitis

Rasmussen's encephalitis is a syndrome with a recently identified autoimmune etiology linked to mechanisms of loss of self-tolerance that may also be important in schizophrenia. Rasmussen's is a rare progressive neurological disease of childhood onset that is characterized by intractable seizures, hemiparesis, and dementia. Recent work by Rogers and colleagues (1994) has linked the pathology in Rasmussen's encephalitis to direct autoantibody stimulation of the glutamate receptor. Homology between this receptor and a microbial amino acid binding protein suggests that the autoimmune response in the disorder may result from cross-reactivity between these two antigens. Circulating autoantibodies are hypothesized to gain access to CNS glutamate receptors following focal disruption of the blood–brain barrier after a seizure or head injury, events known to precede the onset of Rasmussen's encephalitis. Subsequent immune-mediated stimulation of the glutamate receptor would cause more seizures and further blood–brain barrier disruption. Until recently, the treatment of Rasmussen's has been limited to hemispherectomy. On the basis of the presumed autoimmune nature of the illness, treatment using plasmapheresis to clear the antibody has been undertaken with success.

Interestingly, increased rates of head injury and obstetric complications are observed in schizophrenia, as has been discussed elsewhere in this book (see Chapter 1, this volume). Head trauma and disruption of the blood–brain barrier such as that putatively initiating autoimmune pathology in Rasmussen's could theoretically trigger immune-mediated disease in schizophrenia.

Autoantibody Studies in Schizophrenia

The many similarities between known or suspected autoimmune disorders and schizophrenia have stimulated work by our group on autoantibodies to neuronal antigens in patients with schizophrenia. A review of the history of studies of autoantibodies in schizophrenia provides important background.

The search for serum antibrain autoantibodies in schizophrenia has yielded intriguing but controversial results (Knight et al. 1987) that have been difficult to replicate (Ehrnst et al. 1982). Heath and Krupp (1967) conducted a well-known series of studies using immunofluorescence techniques in which they provided evidence for the binding of a circulating factor called "taraxein" to antigens in the region of the septal nuclei. Further evidence of this factor was obtained by injecting serum from healthy control subjects and schizophrenic patients into monkeys. Injection of serum from patients caused behavioral and electroencephalographic changes not seen after injection of serum from control subjects. However, Heath and Krupp's reports have been widely disputed on methodological grounds (Whittingham et al. 1968). Using a radiofixation assay, Baron and colleagues (1977) found higher levels of serum autoantibodies capable of fixation to human brain sections in schizophrenic patients compared with control subjects. Pandey and co-workers (1981), using a hemagglutinin assay, determined that nearly half of a sample of schizophrenic patients but none of a control group had serum or cerebrospinal fluid (CSF) autoantibodies. DeLisi (1986) found that 18% of serum samples of psychiatric patient had autoantibodies. However, this finding was not specific to the schizophrenic patients. Shima and colleagues (1991), using an indirect immunofluorescence method, demonstrated a pattern of antibody binding to CNS tissue that was consistent with nerve cell staining in 27.3% of schizophrenic patients compared with only 1.9% of depressed patients and 0% of healthy control subjects. Furthermore, numerous studies in recent years have demonstrated increased levels of autoantibodies to non-neuronal tissues in schizophrenic patients. Such findings are cited as evidence of nonspecific autoimmune activation in patients with schizophrenia. However, no specific antigens have been identified in this work.

Such findings are difficult to interpret. The fact that autoantibodies are found in healthy individuals (Bird 1988) as well as in germ-free experimental animals suggests that autoantibodies may arise spontaneously. Autoantibodies that cross-react with human antigens may also arise in response to invading viral or bacterial antigens but result in no damage or disease. For example, Stefansson and colleagues (1985), using immunoblotting and immunohistochemical methods, found immunoglobulin M (IgM) and immunoglobulin G (IgG) antibodies against a neurofilament protein in 90% of neurologically healthy individuals. Forty-five of 200 neurologically ill patients had antibodies against CNS proteins other than neurofilaments, as compared with 10 of 200 healthy control subjects.

Conversely, failure to detect antibodies is not necessarily evidence against antibody-mediated autoimmunity. More than 10% of myasthenia gravis patients with severe generalized weakness have no detectable anti–acetylcholine receptor antibodies (Drachman 1990). Knight (1985) argues that commonly employed methods may be insensitive to functional interactions between antibodies and antigens. The use of postmortem tissues may also afford limited ability to detect subtle allosteric interactions between an autoantibody and a cell-surface component.

Studies at Columbia University and New York State Psychiatric Institute

To investigate the specificity of antibodies to neural cells, we tested medically healthy hospitalized patients with schizophrenia or schizoaffective disorder and medical, neurological, and healthy control subjects for the presence of serum antibodies to neuronal proteins. We found that 14 of 32 (44%) patients with schizophrenia had serum IgG antibodies that bound to a human neuroblastoma cell protein of 60 kD molecular weight on Western blot (Kilidireas et al. 1992). Partial sequence analysis of this antigen identified it as the 60-kD heat shock protein (hsp60). Antibodies to hsp60 were detected in only 8 of the 100 control subjects. Additional studies have supported the association of anti-hsp60 antibodies and schizophrenia.

Expression and Purification of hsp60

In the preliminary initial study described above, hsp60 was obtained from cultured neuroblastoma cells and purified by repeated cycles of separation by sodium dodecyl sulfate–polyacrylamide gel electrophoresis. This method was time-consuming, yielded only modest amounts of protein, and involved the risk that co-migrating proteins would not be properly eliminated. In light of these limitations, affinity-purified recombinant hsp60 (rhsp60) was generated in our laboratory and used in subsequent studies. Interpretation of anti-hsp60 reactivity was appreciably easier and more accurate when rhsp60 was used as an antigen.

Confirmation of the Association of Anti-hsp60 Antibodies With Schizophrenia

To confirm the pilot data generated using neuroblastoma cell extracts, we used Western blot analysis to test the reactivity of patient and control serum to 5 µg of rhsp60 at dilutions of 1:1,000, 1:4,000, and 1:10,000. Results of this study of patients with schizophrenia compared with medical, psychiatric, and healthy control subjects confirmed our previous results. At serum dilutions of 1:10,000, anti-hsp60 antibodies were present in 13 of 40 (32.5%) patients with schizophrenia, in 6 of 30 (20%) patients with rheumatological and infectious illness (tuberculosis), but in none of 97 control subjects with no illness, with other nonpsychotic psychiatric illness, or with neurological disease (Table 9–2; Figure 9–2).

hsp60 Autoantibodies in Twin Pairs

Reactivity to rhsp60 was also measured in serum from monozygotic twin pairs discordant and concordant for schizophrenia (serum was provided by Dr. E. Fuller Torrey's sample from the National Institute of Mental Health [NIMH] Neuroscience Center at St. Elizabeth's Hospital) (Table 9–3). Anti-hsp60 antibody was not present in serum from the three pairs of twins concordant for schizophrenia. In the discordant twin sample, we detected hsp60 antibodies in the affected twin (but not the healthy twin) in 5 of the 8 twin pairs studied. Overall, 6 of 16 (37.5%) affected twins were hsp60-antibody positive compared with 2 of 16 (12.5%) unaffected twins. These frequencies are similar to those observed in the population presented in Table 9–2. I discuss the significance of the findings in the twin samples later in this chapter.

Table 9–2. Percentage of subjects in various diagnostic categories with antibodies to hsp60 in serial dilutions

Diagnosis	N	Negative	1:1,000	1:4,000	1:10,000
			% (n)		
Schizophrenia	40	42.5 (17)	57.5 (23)	42.5 (17)	32.5 (13)
Schizoaffective disorder	12	50 (6)	50 (6)	25 (3)	25 (3)
Other psychotic disorder	6	66 (4)	33 (2)	17 (1)	17 (1)
Other nonpsychotic psychiatric disorder	48	46 (22)	44 (26)	10 (5)	0 (0)
Neurological disease	33	88 (29)	12 (4)	3 (1)	0 (0)
Rheumatological disease	20	60 (12)	40 (8)	30 (6)	20 (4)
Tuberculosis	10	50 (5)	50 (5)	30 (3)	20 (2)
Healthy	16	87 (14)	13 (2)	0 (0)	0 (0)

Note. hsp60 = 60-kD heat shock protein.

hsp60, Infection, Autoimmunity, and the Pathophysiology of Schizophrenia

To our knowledge, the finding of antibody reactivity to hsp60 in schizophrenic patients represents the first identification of a putative autoantigen in the illness. To consider the significance of antibodies to hsp60 in the pathophysiology of schizophrenia, it is necessary to understand the role of hsp60 in normal and disease states and its relevance to infection and autoimmune processes in general.

Heat Shock Proteins, Infection, and Autoimmunity

Heat shock proteins have been of great interest to immunologists because of significant sequence homology between heat shock proteins from widely divergent species, including infectious organisms. Antibodies raised against foreign heat shock proteins could give rise to autoimmune reactivity to native heat shock proteins and result in disease or dysfunction via molecular mimicry. The observed reactivity to hsp60 seen in some patients with tuberculosis

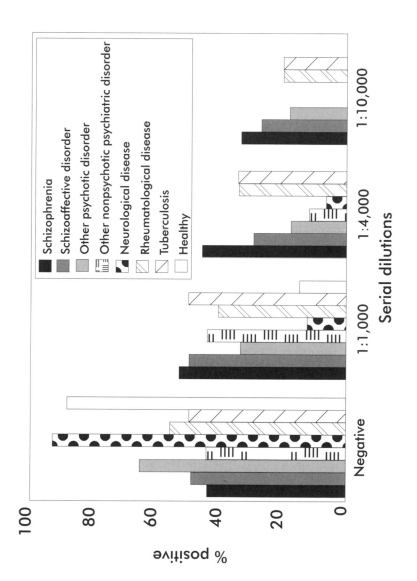

Figure 9–2. Antibodies to recombinant 60-kD heat shock protein (hsp60).

Table 9–3. Presence of hsp60 antibodies in monozygotic twin pairs discordant for schizophrenia[a]

	Twin pairs							
	1	2	3	4	5	6	7	8
Affected twin	+	+	+	+	+	+	–	–
Healthy twin	–	–	–	–	–	+	+	–

Note. hsp60 = 60-kD heat shock protein. + = hsp60 antibody positive; – = hsp60 antibody negative. [a]Six of 6 monozygotic twins concordant for schizophrenia were hsp60 antibody negative.

or autoimmune illness may arise as a result of a structural feature (an *epitope*) recognized by the antibody on both human hsp60 and the bacterial analogue of hsp60; hsp60 is approximately 50% homologous with the 65-kD mycobacterial heat shock protein (hsp65) (Jindal et al. 1989). Human antigens that are cross-reactive with hsp65 have been implicated in the pathogenesis of adjuvant-induced arthritis in rats and of autoimmune diabetes in humans and mice (Elias et al. 1990; Van Eden et al. 1987). In adjuvant-induced arthritis, a proteoglycan link protein is the presumed antigen for cross-reacting anti-hsp65 antibodies (Van Eden et al. 1985).

Biological Role of Heat Shock Proteins

Heat shock proteins are cellular chaperonins that are constitutively expressed in all cells and that function in protein assembly and transport. They are induced in response to a variety of stressful stimuli, including infection, toxins, and cytokine activation. Under conditions of cellular stress, heat shock proteins function to maintain cellular integrity (Lindquist 1986; Morimoto et al. 1994). In humans, for example, heat shock proteins may aid in the recovery from myocardial infarction, surgery, and stroke (Black and Lucchesi 1993; Mestrill and Dillmann 1995). The experimental induction of heat shock proteins has been shown to protect organs and tissues exposed to environmental insults. For example, Tytell and colleagues (1993) examined the protective effects of 70-kD heat shock protein (hsp70) proteins in the retinal cells of albino rats exposed to damage from bright lights. Injection of purified hsp70 reduces photoreceptor cell damage from prolonged light exposure. Similar protection results from the application of a mild heat stress, which similarly induces heat shock proteins.

hsp60 Antibodies and the Pathophysiology of Schizophrenia

Antibodies to heat shock protein in high titer do not occur in healthy individuals, although they are found in a small number of patients with rheumatological and infectious disease such as tuberculosis (Jarjour et al. 1991). In our work, however, schizophrenic patients without clinical or laboratory evidence of medical illness have the highest frequency of anti-hsp60 antibody reactivity.

Antibodies to hsp60 could arise in schizophrenia in genetically susceptible individuals as a result of infection with an organism that contains antigens homologous to hsp60, via molecular mimicry. Alternatively, viral infection could result in the incorporation of hsp60 into the budding virus, making the protein immunogenic. Finally, hsp60 could become immunogenic because of structural alterations or posttranslational modifications secondary to mutation, metabolic changes, or infection (Shattner and Rager-Zisman 1990).

hsp60 antibodies could be related to disease in schizophrenia if they interact with normal or aberrantly produced hsp60 in neuronal cells. Antibodies against hsp60 or subtypes of hsp60 (of either genetic or viral etiology) might directly interfere with the neuronal stress response (see Figure 9–3), and certain neuronal populations could thereby be left vulnerable to fever, infection, head injury, or oxidative stress. Alternatively, aberrant production of hsp60 as a result of mutation or viral modification could similarly impair the ability of certain neuronal populations to respond to environmental stress (see Figure 9–4A). Cellular damage or dysfunction during development or later could give rise to structural or functional abnormalities leading to schizophrenia. Finally, autoantibodies to hsp60 may be markers of neuronal damage rather than causes of such damage. In this scenario, cellular damage and/or disruption of the blood–brain barrier might expose hsp60 to immune surveillance and initiate an autoimmune response (see Figure 9–4B). Alternatively, it is possible that the disease process could involve a physiologically important but as-yet-unidentified neuronal antigen that merely cross-reacts with hsp60.

Cytokines, Autoimmunity, and Schizophrenia

The cytokines may provide another line of evidence linking immune activation, such as that seen in autoimmunity and infection, and schizophrenia. Cytokines are a functionally diverse group of soluble polypeptide hormones with homeostatic and regulatory functions in the immune system. Overexpression of cytokines such as interleukin-1 (IL1), interleukin-2 (IL2), and interleukin-6 (IL6) is seen in human autoimmune diseases (Capra et al. 1990; Greenberg et al. 1988; Halper 1991; Linker-Israeli et al. 1991; Nakanishi et al. 1990; Wood et al. 1988). Similar elevations in plasma and CSF levels of IL1, IL2, and IL6 and aberrant mitogen-induced production of IL2 have been demonstrated in patients with schizophrenia; these findings support autoimmune theories of the disorder (Ganguli et al. 1994; Katila et al. 1994; Licinio et al. 1989; Maes et al. 1994; Rappaport et al. 1989; Shintani et al. 1991; Villemain et al. 1987, 1989; Wei et al. 1992; Xu et al. 1994).

Cytokines including IL1 and IL6 have also been shown to exert wide-ranging direct effects on neuronal populations in vitro and in vivo; both neurotoxic and neuroprotective effects have been ob-

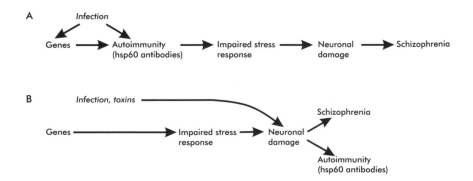

Figure 9–3. Hypothesized mechanisms of genetic/infectious induction of 60-kD heat shock protein (hsp60) in schizophrenia and autoimmune disease.

served. Such research has stimulated active investigation of the role of cytokines in CNS disease. Several findings are of particular relevance to schizophrenia. For example, Denicoff and colleagues (1987), in studies of the behavioral and psychological sequelae of treatment with IL2 in cancer patients, demonstrated that IL2 frequently induces psychosis and other significant neurobehavioral changes. Cytokines can also induce disruption of the blood–brain barrier, thereby indirectly enhancing CNS exposure to the action of circulating immune factors. Finally, it is noteworthy that the hippocampus, which may be anatomically and functionally relevant to the clinical pathology of schizophrenia, is particularly vulnerable to the cytotoxic effects of cytokines. These observations suggest that overexpression of cytokines in schizophrenia may derive from ongoing immune or autoimmune activity, but also that such overexpression may represent evidence of cell injury or may itself be responsible for neuronal injury or dysfunction.

Future Directions

Schizophrenia is an etiologically heterogeneous syndrome, and such heterogeneity adds complexity to and confounds neurobiological investigation of the disorder. In the search for abnormal immune or immune-related mechanisms of disease, it is likely that only a minority of patients would manifest the relevant immune pathophysiology. Our current research efforts therefore seek to better define a subgroup of patients—for example, those with demonstrated hsp60 autoantibodies—in whom further studies of pathophysiology (e.g., studies of cytokines) or environmental exposure (e.g., histories of head trauma, viral exposure, obstetric complications) can be undertaken. Clinical data collection using flexible symptom sets and evaluation of findings according to broad domains of psychopathology may increase the likelihood of defining a clinical subtype in which immune abnormalities contribute to cause or course of illness (Carpenter and Buchanan 1989; Nurnberger et al. 1994). Finally, immune studies in patients with schizophrenia from families with classical autoimmune disorders may help characterize an autoimmune subgroup of patients in whom subtle immunological changes may be identified.

Examination of the relative contributions of genetic vulnerability and environmental insult in a putative "autoimmune subtype" of schizophrenia represents another important direction for future work. It is interesting to speculate, for example, that our studies of a small sample of monozygotic twin pairs suggest that affected discordant twin pairs share a form of schizophrenia in which an immune response (e.g., to a virus) exerts a major and predominant effect on disease development. In contrast, in the concordant monozygotic twin pairs, genetic influence alone could be sufficient for disease expression. Family genetic studies of autoantibody production and studies of environmental exposures in patients with identified autoimmune pathology may help clarify this relationship.

Longitudinal studies of aberrant immune measures may help define state versus trait contributions to observed aberrant immune measures. For example, a correlation of hsp60 antibody titers with acute psychopathological change in schizophrenia would indicate that antibodies reflect an active disease process and do not merely constitute markers of remote injury, such as that which might occur during development.

Immune studies in larger and independent samples are needed, given that our work to date is potentially confounded by sample size and selection limitations as well as limitations in the adequacy of the "controls" used. For example, hospitalized patients with schizophrenia may differ from neurological, healthy, and nonpsychotic psychiatric control subjects in terms of a range of environmental exposures (including medication treatment) that could result in antibody production but be unrelated to disease.

In the laboratory, epitope-mapping studies may help elucidate and characterize an hsp60 antibody binding site recognized by antibodies from patients with schizophrenia that is distinct from the sites recognized by antibodies from control subjects. Efforts to identify cross-reactive epitopes from viral and other infectious agents may help to shed light on the relationship of anti-hsp60 antibodies to prior infection and may stimulate investigations of the role of such an agent in the pathology of schizophrenia. Epitope-mapping analysis will permit identification of other functionally important cross-reacting proteins that may be relevant to the disease process. The hypothesis that hsp60 may be aberrantly expressed, altered, or distributed in the brains of patients with schizophrenia will be tested using immunohistochemical techniques on postmortem tissue. Clinical and laboratory work will be undertaken to examine the relationship of hsp60 autoantibody and cytokine production in patients and control subjects.

Conclusion

The immune system is now known to exert diverse effects on the CNS in health and in disease. Autoimmune mechanisms have been identified in a range of CNS disease states; the presumed etiological influences, pathophysiological processes, and clinical features of these syndromes share important characteristics with schizophrenia.

Our group has demonstrated abnormal autoantibodies to a CNS stress protein, hsp60, in a subgroup of patients with schizophrenia. Although these findings require replication, it is intriguing to speculate that aberrantly produced or modified hsp60, or antibodies to hsp60, could be involved in the pathophysiology of the disorder by impairing neuronal response to stressors such as infection, fever, toxins, or trauma or by other mechanisms. Alternatively, such autoantibodies may be secondary to and serve as markers of neuronal injury from other causes. Similarly, cytokines, which are believed to mediate neuronal response to stress, are observed to be overexpressed in schizophrenia and may themselves directly or indirectly cause neuronal injury, impair neuronal function, or serve as markers of such changes (Figure 9–4).

Whether hsp60 antibodies and cytokine abnormalities are causally related to the pathology of schizophrenia or represent secondary responses to neuronal injury is the fundamental question requiring further investigation. Certainly, the identification of specific immune-mediated mechanisms in schizophrenia would sug-

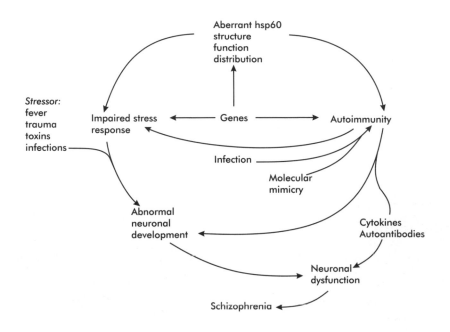

Figure 9–4. Summary of interrelationships between autoimmunity, genes, neuronal function, and schizophrenia. hsp60 = 60-kD heat shock protein.

gest new therapeutic strategies aimed at interfering with antibody and cytokine action or modifying cellular vulnerability to injury.

References

Baron M, Stern M, Anavi R, et al: Tissue binding factor in schizophrenic sera: a clinical and genetic study. Biol Psychiatry 12:199–219, 1977

Bird G: Autoantibodies—a perspective, in B Lymphocytes in Human Disease. Edited by Bird G, Calvert JA. London, Oxford University Press, 1978, pp 409–424

Black SC, Lucchesi BR: Heat shock, proteins and the ischemic heart: an endogenous protective mechanism. Circulation 87:1048–1051, 1993

Bonfa E, Golombek SJ, Kaufman LD, et al: Association between lupus psychosis and anti-ribosomal P protein antibodies. N Engl J Med 317: 265–271, 1987

Capra R, Mattioli F, Marciano N, et al: Significantly higher levels of soluble interleukin-2 in patients with relapsing-remitting multiple sclerosis compared with healthy subjects (letter). Arch Neurol 47:254, 1990

Carpenter WT Jr, Buchanan RW: Domains of psychopathology relevant to the study of etiology and treatment in schizophrenia, in Schizophrenia: Scientific Progress. Edited by Schulz SC. New York, Oxford University Press, 1989, pp 13–22

Cohen IR: A heat shock protein, molecular mimicry and autoimmunity. Isr J Med Sci 26:673–676, 1990

Crow TJ: Is schizophrenia an infectious disease? Lancet 1:173–175, 1983

DeLisi LE: Neuroimmunology: clinical studies of schizophrenia and other psychiatric disorders, in Handbook of Schizophrenia, Vol 1: The Neurology of Schizophrenia. Edited by Nasrallah HA, Weinberger DR. New York, Elsevier, 1986, pp 377–396

Denicoff KD, Rubinow DR, Papa MZ, et al: The neuropsychiatric effects of treatment with interleukin-2 and lymphokine-activated killer cells. Ann Intern Med 107:293–300, 1987

Drachman DB: How to recognize an antibody mediated autoimmune disease criteria, in Immunologic Mechanisms in Neurologic and Psychiatric Disease. Edited by Waksman BH. New York, Raven, 1990, pp 183–186

Ehrnst A, Wiesel FK, Bjerkenstedt L, et al: Failure to detect immunologic stigmata in schizophrenia. Neuropsychobiology 8:169–171, 1982

Elias D, Markovits D, Reshef T, et al: Induction and therapy of autoimmune diabetes in the non-obese diabetic (NOD/Lt) mouse by a k5kDa heat shock protein. Proc Natl Acad Sci U S A 87:1576–1580, 1990

Gahring LC, Twyman RE, Greenlee JE, et al: Autoantibodies to neuronal glutamate receptors in patients with paraneoplastic neurodegenerative syndrome enhance receptor activation. Mol Med 1:245–253, 1995

Ganguli R, Yang A, Shurin G, et al: Serum interleukin-6 concentration in schizophrenia: elevation associated with duration of illness. Psychiatry Res 51:1–10, 1994

Greenberg SJ, Marcon L, Hurwitz BJ, et al: Elevated levels of soluble interleukin-2 receptors in multiple sclerosis. N Engl J Med 319:1019–1020, 1988

Halper J: Immunocyte receptors and second messengers in psychoneuro-immunology, in Psychoimmunology Update. Edited by Gorman JG, Kertzner RM. Washington, DC, American Psychiatric Press, 1991, pp 113–151

Heath RG, Krupp IM: Schizophrenia as an immunologic disorder I, II, III. Arch Gen Psychiatry 16:1–33, 1967

Husby G, van de Rijn I, Zabriskie JB, et al: Antibodies reacting with cytoplasm of subthalamic and caudate nuclei neurons in chorea and acute rheumatic fever. J Exp Med 144:1094–1110, 1976

Jarjour WN, Jeffried BD, Davies JS, et al: Autoantibodies to human stress proteins. Arthritis Rheum 34:1133–1138, 1991

Jindal S, Dudani AK, Singh B, et al: Primary structure of a human mitochondrial protein homologous to the bacterial and plant chaperonins and to the 65 kD mycobacterial antigen. Molecular Cell Biology 9: 2279–2283, 1989

Katila H, Hurme M, Wahlbeck K, et al: Plasma and cerebrospinal fluid interleukin-1 and interleukin-6 in hospitalized schizophrenic patients. Neuropsychobiology 30:20–23, 1994

Kiessling LS, Marcotte AC, Culpepper L: Antineuronal antibodies in movement disorders. Pediatrics 92:39–43, 1993

Kilidireas K, Latov N, Strauss DH, et al: Antibodies to the human 60 kDa heat-shock protein in patients with schizophrenia. Lancet 340:569–572, 1992

Knight JG: Possible autoimmune mechanisms in schizophrenia. Integrative Psychiatry 3:134–143, 1985

Knight JG, Knight A, Pert CB: Is schizophrenia really a virally triggered antireceptor autoimmune disease? in Biological Perspectives on Schizophrenia. Edited by Helmchen HJ, Henn FA. New York, Wiley, 1987, pp 107–124

Licinio J, Krystal JH, Seibyl JP, et al: Elevated central levels of interleukin-2 in drug free schizophrenia patients (abstract). Schizophr Res 4:372, 1991

Lindquist S: The heat shock proteins. Annu Rev Biochem 55:1151–1191, 1986

Linker-Israeli M, Deans RJ, Wallace DJ, et al: Elevated levels of endogenous IL6 in systemic lupus erythematosus: a putative role in pathogenesis. J Immunol 147:117–123, 1991

Maes M, Meltzer HY, Bosmans E: Immune-inflammatory markers in schizophrenia: comparison to normal controls and effects of clozapine. Acta Psychiatr Scand 89:346–351, 1994

Mednick SA, Machon RA, Huttunen MO, et al: Adult schizophrenia following prenatal exposure to an influenza epidemic. Arch Gen Psychiatry 45:189–192, 1988

Mestrill R, Dillmann WH: Heat shock proteins and protection against myocardial ischemia. J Mol Cell Cardiol 27:45–52, 1995

Morimoto RI, Tissieres A, Georgopoulos C: The Biology of Heat Shock Proteins and Molecular Chaperones. Cold Spring Harbor, NY, Cold Spring Harbor Laboratory Press, 1994

Naidu S, Narasimhachari N: Sydenham's chorea: a possible presynaptic dopaminergic dysfunction initially. Ann Neurol 8:445–446, 1980

Nakanishi K, Malek TR, Smith KA, et al: Both interleukin-2 and a second T cell derived factor in EL4 supernatants have activity as differentiation factors in IgM synthesis. J Exp Med 160:1605–1621, 1990

Nausieda PA, Bieliauskas LA, Bacon LD, et al: Chronic dopaminergic sensitivity after Sydenham's chorea. Neurology 33:750–754, 1983

Newsome-Davis J: Lambert Eaton myasthenic syndrome. Monogr Allergy 25:116–124, 1988

Nurnberger JI Jr, Blehar MC, Kaufmann CA, et al: Diagnostic interview for genetic studies: rationale, unique features and training. Arch Gen Psychiatry 51:849–859, 1994

Pandey RS, Gutpa AK, Chaturvedi VC: Autoimmune model of schizophrenia with special reference to antibrain antibodies. Biol Psychiatry 16:1123–1136, 1981

Rappaport MH, McAllister CG, Pickar D, et al: Elevated levels of interleukin-2 receptors in schizophrenia. Arch Gen Psychiatry 46:291–292, 1989

Richman DP, Fairclough RH, Xu Q, et al: Noninflammatory immune mechanisms in disease of the nervous system, in Immunologic Mechanisms in Neurologic and Psychiatric Disease. Edited by Waksman BH. New York, Raven, 1990, pp 55–65

Rogers SW, Andrews PI, Gahring LC, et al: Autoantibodies to glutamate receptor GluR3 in Rasmussen's encephalitis. Science 265:648–651, 1994

Shattner A, Rager-Zisman B: Virus-induced autoimmunity. Reviews of Infectious Diseases 12:204–222, 1990

Shima S, Yano K, Sugiura M, et al: Anticerebral antibodies in functional psychoses. Biol Psychiatry 29:322–328, 1991

Shintani F, Kanba S, Maruo N, et al: Serum interleukin-6 in schizophrenic patients. Life Sci 49:661–664, 1991

Sinha AA, Lopez MR, McDevitt HO: Autoimmune diseases: the failure of self-tolerance. Science 248:1380–1388, 1990

Smith BR, McLachlin SM, Furmaniak J: Autoantibodies to the thyrotropin receptor. Endocr Rev 9:106–121, 1988

Solimena M, Folli F, Aparisi R, et al: Autoantibodies to GABA-ergic neurons and pancreatic beta cells in stiff-man syndrome. N Engl J Med 322:1555–1560, 1990

Stefansson K, Marton LS, Dieperink ME: Circulating antibodies to the 200 kD protein of neurofilaments in the serum of healthy individuals. Science 228:1117–1119, 1985

Strauss DH, Printz DJ: Autoimmune phenomena, neuronal stress, and schizophrenia, in Schizophrenia: New Directions for Clinical Research and Treatment. Edited by Kaufmann CA, Gorman JM. New York, Mary Ann Liebert, 1996, pp 137–152

Swedo SE, Leonard HL, Schapiro MB, et al: Sydenham's chorea: physical and psychological symptoms of St Vitus dance. Pediatrics 91:706–713, 1993

Tytell M, Barbe MF, Brown IR: Stress (heat shock) protein accumulation in the central nervous system: its relationship to cell stress and damage. Adv Neurol 59:293–303, 1993

Van Eden W, Holoshitz J, Nevo Z, et al: Arthritis induced by a T-lymphocyte clone that responds to mycobacteria tuberculosis and to cartilage proteoglycan. Proc Natl Acad Sci U S A 82:5117–5120, 1985

Van Eden W, Holoshitz J, Cohen IR: Antigen mimicry between mycobacterial and cartilage proteoglycans: the model of adjuvant arthritis. Concepts Immunopathol 4:144–170, 1987

Villemain F, Chatenoud L, Guillibert E, et al: Decreased production of interleukin-2 in schizophrenia. Ann N Y Acad Sci 496:669–675, 1987

Villemain F, Chatenoud L, Galinowsky A, et al: Aberrant T cell–mediated immunity in untreated schizophrenic patients: deficient interleukin-2 production. Am J Psychiatry 146:609–616, 1989

Wang S, Sun CE, Walczak CA, et al: Evidence for a susceptibility locus for schizophrenia on chromosome 6pter–p22. Nat Genet 10:41–46, 1995

Wei J, Xu H, Davies JL, et al: Increase of plasma IL-6 concentration with age in health subjects. Life Sci 51:1953–1956, 1992

Wilcox JA, Nasrallah HA: Sydenham's chorea and psychosis. Neuro-psychobiology 15:13–14, 1986

Wilcox JA, Nasrallah HA: Sydenham's chorea and psychopathology. Neuropsychobiology 19:6–8, 1988

Whittingham S, Mackay IR, Jones IH, et al: Absence of brain antibodies in patients with schizophrenia (abstract). BMJ 1:347, 1968

Wong DF, Wagner HN Jr, Tune LE, et al: Positron emission tomography reveals elevated D_2 receptors in drug-naive schizophrenics. Science 234:1558–1563, 1986

Wood NC, Symons JA, Duff GW: Serum interleukin-2 receptor in rheumatoid arthritis: a prognostic indicator of disease activity? J Autoimmun 1:353–361, 1988

Wright P, Murray RM: Schizophrenia: prenatal influenza and autoimmunity. Ann Med 25:497–502, 1993

Xu HM, Wei J, Hemmings GP: Changes of plasma concentrations of interleukin-1a and interleukin-6 with neuroleptic treatment for schizophrenia. Br J Psychiatry 164:251–253, 1994

Zinkernagel RM, Cooper S, Chambers J, et al: Virus-induced autoantibody response to a transgenic viral antigen. Nature 345:68–71, 1990

Conclusion

Schizophrenia—Closing the Gap Between Genetics, Epidemiology, and Prevention

Richard Jed Wyatt, M.D.

The primary goal of genetic and epidemiological research in schizophrenia is to prevent the disorder. There have traditionally been three types of prevention: primary, secondary, and tertiary (Jamison 1993). For schizophrenia, primary prevention aims to decrease the incidence of the illness by reducing its risk factors or by instituting policies to forestall its emergence. Secondary prevention aims to reduce schizophrenia's duration or severity or to reduce physiological and psychosocial risk factors that would lead to further adverse consequences. Secondary prevention also encompasses the possibility of a cure, which, by definition, can only occur once the disorder has begun. Tertiary prevention includes rehabilitation aimed at restoring or partially restoring the lost function resulting from a previous or ongoing illness. Tertiary prevention also includes palliative measures to reduce pain and suffering when a cure or rehabilitation is not available. Dividing the above measures into three categories under the larger rubric of prevention is conceptually awkward and may have outlived its usefulness (Marzek and Haggerty 1994); nevertheless, the three divisions provide a simple framework for considering the topics raised in this book.

During the 1950s and 1960s, attempts at primary prevention of

The author is grateful to Ioline Henter for her excellent editorial assistance.

schizophrenia in the United States were led by the community mental health movement. These prevention efforts were essentially psychological and educational; unfortunately, they did not work. Furthermore, any success they might have achieved could not be measured, because no system had been instituted to demonstrate change in incidence rates. In addition, the community mental health movement lacked the knowledge to design workable interventions (Wyatt 1985). Another significant failure of the movement was that its services were usually physically and theoretically detached from the settings in which individuals with schizophrenia resided and in which the illness was most likely to develop. Schizophrenia is most common in lower socioeconomic classes of the inner cities (Dohrenwend et al. 1992; Kohn 1976; Wyatt et al. 1988), a group that the community mental health movement usually did not reach.

Despite psychiatry's sometimes clumsy attempts to employ the techniques of primary prevention for schizophrenia, there has been considerable success in reducing the incidence of a number of other illnesses that in the past were misdiagnosed as schizophrenia. The introduction of early treatments for syphilis made general paresis of the insane a rarity; niacin enrichment of whole-grain cereal products has essentially prevented the dementia associated with pellagra; and the use of iodized salt has virtually extinguished the myxedema madness of endemic goiter. Individuals born with inactive phenylalanine hydroxylase were once at risk for developing extreme psychotic states; these individuals can now be diagnosed with prenatal DNA analysis (as well as postnatal biochemical tests) and treated with a low-phenylalanine diet.

This successful treatment of illnesses often mistaken for schizophrenia was, and continues to be, a form of primary prevention; however, most of our present targeted interventions for schizophrenia are secondary or tertiary. In contrast, the chapters of this book explore a number of new findings, many of which could strongly affect our current conception of primary intervention for this disorder. In this concluding chapter, I highlight some of these intriguing studies and discuss how the findings could be used to eventually develop preventive measures for schizophrenia.

Links Between Schizophrenia and Maternal/Fetal Immunological Incompatibilities

Hollister and Brown, in Chapter 8 of this volume, describe a condition that has not been previously recognized as producing schizophrenia—Rhesus (Rh) incompatibility. Rh incompatibility is associated with hemolytic disease of the newborn (HDN), which the authors believe to be the most likely etiological factor. Of the five major antigens in the Rh system, the D antigen is the most immunogenic and is the most common cause of HDN. Rh HDN is a disorder associated with anemia, hepatomegaly, hypoxia, hyperbilirubinemia, and a variety of symptoms, many involving the central nervous system (CNS). It occurs when the Rh-positive erythrocytes of a fetus are exposed to immunoglobulin G (IgG) antibodies from a previously sensitized Rh-negative mother. Apparently, those infants who survive HDN without experiencing severe neurological deficits are at risk for developing schizophrenia. If the association between Rh incompatibility and schizophrenia is confirmed, it will be a further reason to ensure that HDN is prevented. In the United States, most, but not all, women with Rh-incompatible pregnancies are treated immediately after delivery with RhD immune globulin (anti-D gamma globulin prophylaxis [Rhogam]) to prevent HDN in subsequent births.

HDN is a multifactorial disorder as defined by Malaspina, Sohler, and Susser in Chapter 2 of this volume; it occurs because of the coming together during a pregnancy of specific antigens (or the absence of an antigen for Rh-negative individuals) produced by the Rh gene or genes in a previously sensitized woman and her fetus. While it is relatively common for Caucasians to be either Rh-positive or Rh-negative, the number of Rh-positive individuals is almost six-fold greater than that of Rh-negative individuals. In addition, in Rh HDN, it is the Rh-positive fetus who is affected. If schizophrenia is indeed associated with the most abundant variant (Rh-positive), it differs from most classical genetic diseases, in which the responsible genes occur in only a relatively small percentage of the population. At a time when we are on the verge of mapping the entire genome and are expecting to derive enormous benefits from that knowledge, it is important to emphasize that for many psychiatric disorders, it will probably be the interaction of the gene or genes with the environment that will be found to be responsible for the illness. Multifactorial disorders require an understanding beyond that which can be derived from molecular genetics alone (Prescott and Gottesman 1993; Strohman 1994; Wyatt 1996).

The apparent association between Rh HDN and the development of schizophrenia should kindle interest in other maternal–fetal immunological incompatibilities, and ABO incompatibility in particular. ABO incompatibility occurs in about 20% of pregnancies, and the jaundice that accompanies it is milder and less common than that accompanying Rh incompatibility. ABO incompatibility occurs when a woman with type O blood carries a fetus with either type A or type B blood. Type O individuals carry no A or B antigens on their erythrocytes and thus can be universal donors for blood transfusions. However, they can become exposed to A and B antigens that are present in many other species, including the normal flora of the gastrointestinal system, and thus become sensitized (readily make antibodies) to those antigens. Blood type A and B individuals make antibodies to the reciprocal antigen (A to B and B to A), but these are immunoglobulin M (IgM) antibodies that do not cross the placenta and destroy fetal erythrocytes.

It has been known for some time, although perhaps not widely, that individuals with schizophrenia have a slightly higher than expected rate of type B blood (Mourant et al. 1978), although additional epidemiological studies are needed to determine whether type O mother/type A or B fetus dyads are also increased in schizophrenia. If an increased rate of such pregnancies is found to be associated with schizophrenia, it will also be important to determine the degree of erythrocyte hemolysis necessary to damage the brain and produce schizophrenia. ABO incompatibility represents a spectrum of hemolytic disease, ranging from hemolysis with little laboratory evidence of erythrocyte sensitization to severe hemolytic disease with clear evidence of erythrocyte sensitization (Desjardins et al. 1979). Hollister and Brown's findings (see Chapter 8, this volume) on Rh-incompatible pregnancies suggest that it may be important to focus greater attention on ABO-incompatible pregnancies than has previously seemed necessary.

Links Between Schizophrenia and Influenza

In Chapter 4, Wright and colleagues discuss the apparent association between influenza infection during the second trimester of pregnancy and subsequent development of schizophrenia in the offspring of infected mothers. They argue that because studies have consistently replicated the finding that the influenza virus is associated with schizophrenia, nonspecific factors such as cytokines, which occur with many infections, are unlikely to be the teratogenic agents. They further reason that because the influenza virus probably does not enter the fetal circulation, the virus itself is not likely to be teratogenic. Wright et al. propose that it is a maternal antibody to the influenza virus that constitutes an etiological risk factor for schizophrenia; they call their proposal the "teratogenic antibody hypothesis."

Although the placenta is designed to protect the fetus from some maternal toxins, including most antibodies, IgG antibodies are transferred across the placenta by fraction crystallizable (Fc) binding to specific receptors on the trophoblastic cells. At birth, these antibodies protect the infant against infections until it can make its own IgG antibodies. Because IgG antibodies are the only ones to readily cross the placenta, the influenza antibody implicated in Wright and colleagues' hypothesis would be an IgG antibody.

It may be of some importance to the teratogenic antibody hypothesis that IgG serum influenza antibodies peak between 21 and 49 days after the onset of the disease and probably remain at relatively high titers for a number of months (Couch 1993; Gresser and Halstead 1959; Murphy et al. 1982). Because schizophrenia has only been associated with influenza infection that occurs during the second trimester, the delay and extended period of peak antibody titers would focus attention on the late second, or, more likely, the third trimester as the time when fetal damage is most likely to occur.

In Chapter 3, Nowakowski describes three stages of CNS development in which neurons or glia might be altered on their way to becoming mature cells: cell proliferation, neuronal migration, and neuronal differentiation. These developmental stages continue throughout pregnancy, and a toxic event during any of them could alter the normal development of the CNS. Evidence from autopsy studies (Akbarian et al. 1995; Bogerts 1993; Jakob and Beckmann 1986) indicates that an arrest of normal neuronal migration occurs in schizophrenia; some neurons may not reach their intended targets within the brain. The tenets of the teratogenic antibody hypothesis would suggest that it is the cross-reaction of maternal influenza IgG antibodies and fetal neural elements that alters the migration of these neurons, perhaps during the late second or third trimester, when influenza antibody titers have peaked.

Because schizophrenia has not been associated with other acute infections, Wright and colleagues (Chapter 4, this volume) argue that nonspecific factors associated with infection, such as cytokine production, are not responsible for altering the CNS of the fetus. It may be, however, that other acute febrile infections—for instance, chicken pox or measles—are too rare during pregnancy for an epidemiological link with schizophrenia to be easily established. Thus, while the argument that the teratogenic agent is an antibody to the influenza virus is of great theoretical interest, considerably more information about the nature of the antibody and its cross-reactivity with the developing fetal brain is needed.

Nonetheless, any assumption that the influenza virus, or a pregnant mother's reaction to that virus, is teratogenic would mean that the maternal–fetal immune balance would be disturbed and that the fetus could be seriously affected. Pregnancy is normally a time when women seem to undergo an attenuation of cell-mediated immunity with a concomitant strengthening of antibody-related immunity. For example, systemic lupus erythematosus, which is largely mediated by increased autoantibody production, may flare up during pregnancy. On the other hand, rheumatoid arthritis, which is a cell-mediated autoimmune disorder, often improves during pregnancy (Nelson et al. 1993). This improvement has been related to maternal–fetal disparity (Nelson et al. 1993) of the highly polymorphic immune system–recognition molecule, known as human leukocyte antigen (HLA).

The HLA genotype is highly influential in determining the body's ability to respond to and degree of response to specific antigens, and many of the autoimmune diseases have been found to be associated with specific HLA genotypes. Because repeated studies have shown that rheumatoid arthritis is rare in schizophrenia (Eaton et al. 1992; Vinogradov et al. 1991) and is associated with HLA DR4, Wright and colleagues (see Chapter 4, this volume) examined individuals with schizophrenia for the presence of HLA DR4. As predicted (Knight 1985; Knight et al. 1992), they found a decreased rate of HLA DR4 in patients with schizophrenia as well as in an unrelated sample of the mothers of schizophrenia patients. This finding suggests that something associated with HLA DR4 may make individuals less susceptible to schizophrenia. Significantly, individuals with one autoimmune disease tend to have an excess of other autoimmune diseases, and individuals with HLA DR4 are also at an increased risk for developing insulin-dependent diabetes mellitus (IDDM). Feney (1989) found that individuals with schizophrenia have a decreased incidence of IDDM, which is consistent with their also having a lower rate of HLA DR4 (Feney 1989). In contrast, Wright and colleagues found increased IDDM in the first-degree relatives of schizophrenia patients (they did not study the schizophrenia patients themselves). Why individuals with schizophrenia would have a decreased rate of IDDM when their relatives have an increased rate is unclear. Others, although not consistently, have described a decreased incidence of cancer (Mortensen 1994), certain infections (Carter and Watts 1971), hay fever, asthma (Ehrentheil 1957), and resistance to sensitization by foreign proteins (Molholm 1942) in individuals with schizophrenia.

Thus, it is possible that some aspect of schizophrenia provides broad-spectrum protection against certain other diseases, in particular those that develop before individuals reach reproductive maturity. If schizophrenia does indeed provide such a protective advantage, this could be evidence for the long-sought evolutionary advantage (necessary for any disorder to sustain itself in the population) of schizophrenia (Carter and Watts 1971; Erlenmeyer-Kimling 1968; Huxley et al. 1964). It is more likely that such an advantage would be against infectious agents that perhaps coincide with or precede rheumatoid arthritis and IDDM rather than against these disorders themselves; for example, compared with control children, a high percentage of children with newly diagnosed IDDM have increased titers of antibodies to Coxsackie virus (Clements et al. 1995). If this association proves to be real, it could mean that the genes associated with schizophrenia might protect against Coxsackie or similar viruses. It may also be of interest that two research groups (Kosower et al. 1995; Saha et al. 1990) have reported alterations in the percentages of Duffy blood group antigens in schizophrenia patients compared with healthy control subjects. The authors of these studies suggest that the differences might reflect alterations in other proteins to which the Duffy blood group gene is linked, such as a pseudogene for the D_5 dopamine receptor (Kosower et al. 1995). Significantly, individuals without the usual Duffy blood group antigens [Fy(a⁻b⁻)] are protected from one form of malaria, *Plasmodium vivax (P. vivax)* (Horuk et al. 1993). Most West Africans, or people with origins in that region, have the Duffy-negative Fy phenotype and are therefore resistant to *P. vivax* malaria (White and Breman 1994). This may be similar to the better-known association between sickle-cell anemia and malaria, wherein individuals heterozygous for sickle-cell anemia gain slight protection against *Plasmodium falciparum (P. falciparum)* malaria, the most common form of the disease and the one that causes the most deaths (Bunn 1994).

It is also of some interest that many (Antonarakis et al. 1995; Moises et al. 1995; Schwab et al. 1995; Straub et al. 1995; Wang et al. 1995), but not all, genetic studies of schizophrenia have found a linkage with the short arm of chromosome 6 (chromosome 6p); significantly, this part of the genome also codes for the HLA antigens. Although the linkages do not appear to be to the HLA genes, they are also not far from the HLA loci; thus, they may yet be found to be related to the HLA system.

Finally, in Chapter 5, Brown and Susser review other potential pathways by which prenatal influenza might cause schizophrenia.

They point to variables intervening between the virus and the developing fetus. For instance, there is some evidence that, for pregnant women, one of the side effects of using flu medication may be an increased risk of neural tube defects (Lynberg et al. 1994). Neural tube defects are associated with enlarged ventricles, which have frequently been seen in schizophrenia (Waddington 1993) and have occasionally been shown to be present before the onset of the illness (Weinberger 1988). The fever associated with influenza may also increase rates of neural tube defects (Shiota 1982). Brown and Susser point out that viral infections may produce a vasculitis that can decrease placental circulation, leading to hypoxia of fetal tissues (Catalano and Sever 1971). In this regard, infections such as influenza stimulate T cell lymphocyte production of cytokines. Wegmann and colleagues (1993) have hypothesized that some cytokines (e.g., interleukin-3, granulocyte-macrophage colony-stimulating hormone) promote pregnancy while others (e.g., interleukin-2, interferon gamma, tumor necrosis factor alpha [TNF-α]) can have extremely deleterious effects (Wegmann et al. 1993). Interestingly, the gene for TNF-α is also located on chromosome 6p and is polymorphic. Individuals with the *TNFA2* allele are seven times more likely than those in the general population to develop or die from serious neurological complications of malaria (McGuire et al. 1994). In fact, exposure to malaria, perhaps through the production of cytokines such as TNF-α, appears to provide protection against developing some autoimmune diseases (Knight et al. 1992; Wilson and Duff 1995a, 1995b). Conceivably, this might explain why schizophrenia has repeatedly been found to be less severe in developing countries (Eaton 1991).

Most importantly, Brown and Susser suggest that many of the limitations of earlier investigations of prenatal influenza exposure might be addressed by the Prenatal Determinants of Schizophrenia (PDS) study. The PDS study will review data from almost 12,000 live births from 1959 through 1966 in the Oakland Hospital of the Kaiser Foundation Health Plan; these individuals continued to participate in the Plan through 1981 or later. This cohort has the advantage of being a large and representative sample of births, with a rich array of prospectively collected data pertaining to measures of maternal health, nutrition, use of prescribed and non-prescribed medications, and complications of pregnancy and delivery as well as the availability of stored serum samples from pregnant mothers throughout their gestations. Investigators will be able not only to ascertain influenza exposure from the records but also to document changes in serial antibody titers from the sera, making it possible to identify women who had subsyndromal cases of influenza that would not have been documented in the medical records. Examination of serum titers should also allow investigators to more accurately demonstrate that the reported illness was in fact influenza rather than having to rely on subjective descriptions, and to pinpoint when it occurred.

Another intriguing issue related to the role of influenza infection in schizophrenia is that of nutritional deficiencies. Nutritional deficiencies due to vomiting or loss of appetite through nausea are a possible consequence of influenza. If these symptoms occur in a woman with already poor nutrition, the resulting nutritional deficiencies might be teratogenic. Evidence for the teratogenic effects of extremely poor nutrition comes from studies of the Dutch Hunger Winter (Stein et al. 1975). The Dutch Hunger Winter took place toward the end of the World War II when the Nazis starved part of The Netherlands in retaliation for that country's aid to the Allies, who had just invaded northern Europe. Women who were pregnant during this famine were noted to have an increased number of children with neural tube defects. Hoek and colleagues (Chapter 6 of this volume) describe the original Dutch Famine Study and their further studies with this population (Susser and Lin 1992; Susser et al. 1996). These investigators found that the offspring of mothers who were subjected to this famine during the first trimester of pregnancy had an increased risk of developing schizophrenia. To further underscore the role that nutritional deficiencies might play in the neurodevelopment of schizophrenia, Butler and colleagues (Chapter 7, this volume) describe the ample evidence that normal development of the nervous system does not occur when there has been major nutritional deprivation, and that nutritional deprivation can come from genetic or environmental factors as well as from a combination of the two.

Implications for Prevention

Secondary Prevention

I began this chapter by stating that the primary goal of genetic and epidemiological research in schizophrenia is to prevent the disorder. However, much current research in schizophrenia is aimed at improving rehabilitation for chronically debilitated patients (Liberman and Corrigan 1993). Schizophrenia is an illness that primarily affects individuals in late adolescence and early adulthood, a period when important cognitive, social, and executive skills are developed. Aside from loss of the invaluable period when these skills are ordinarily honed, major rehabilitation efforts are hampered by the continued presence of a thought disorder, extreme distractibility, and, often, significant deficit symptoms. At present, only a limited arsenal of interventions is available to decrease the morbidity of schizophrenia, but some of the available interventions have been instrumental in defining the direction that preventive measures might eventually take. The use of antipsychotic medications, for example, is widely recognized as helpful in decreasing some of schizophrenia's immediate symptoms. Once there is evidence that an individual has schizophrenia, however, is it possible to intervene to prevent a putatively inevitable predetermined outcome? In Chapter 1 of this volume, Waddington and colleagues point out that early, neurodevelopmental origins and later, adult disease progression are *not* mutually exclusive and may be sequential phases of one longitudinal process or separate dimensions of the same pathology. These authors go on to discuss the possibility that the onset of psychosis may reflect an active process which, when unchecked by treatment, links neurodevelopmental disturbances with the progressive increase in morbidity.

In other venues (Davis 1985; Waddington et al. 1995; Wyatt 1991, 1995a, 1995b), it has been argued that secondary prevention during the 1940s and 1950s with convulsive therapies, and during the last 50 years with antipsychotic medications, may have been partially successful in preventing one of the worst forms of the illness—"catastrophic schizophrenia" (Bleuler 1978) or muteness (Waddington et al. 1995). Evidence also exists that early treatment of schizophrenia with antipsychotic medications may prevent some of the long-term morbidity associated with the illness (Wyatt 1991). Just how antipsychotic medications produce this protective effect is unclear. One suggestion is that something about or associated with psychosis is toxic to the brain (Wyatt 1991). There is, however, very little evidence that schizophrenia itself progresses beyond the initial few years or that changes take place in the brain during this time. Strauss, in Chapter 9, discusses his finding of elevated IgG antibody to the 60-kilodalton (kD) heat shock protein (hsp60) in the serum of schizophrenia patients. Although this finding is open to a number of interpretations, one possible explanation is that these autoantibodies may be markers for ongoing neuronal damage. Such damage might be related to some aspect of being psychotic. Strauss points out that cytokines, perhaps released during psychosis, can disrupt the blood–brain barrier and indirectly enhance the CNS's exposure to the action of circulating immune factors. One of the cytokines, interleukin-2, apparently induced psychosis directly when given to patients with cancer (Denicoff et al. 1987). Researchers have also found an increase in the 120-kD band of the neural cell adhesion molecule (N-CAM) in the cerebrospinal fluid (CSF), but not the serum, of patients with chronic schizophrenia, which also suggests an active process of neuronal damage (Poltorak et al. 1995). Finally, still other phase-reactant substances, indicative of an ongoing process, have been found in the CSF of schizophrenia patients (Wiederkehr 1991).

One argument against schizophrenia's being an ongoing process is that there is very little evidence of gliosis, a hallmark of any active inflammatory process. It is, however, now well recognized that neuronal loss can take place in the brain in the absence of gliosis, and, in fact, that such cell loss is a normal part of development and cell pruning (Coyle and Puttfacken 1993; Raff et al. 1993).

Primary Prevention

Although we must continue to search for ways of optimizing treatment for those who already have schizophrenia, it may be time to shift some of our attention and resources to the search for better methods of preventing the illness from developing. As the poet T. S. Eliot wrote,

> [t]he fact that a problem will certainly take a long time to solve, and that it will demand the attention of many minds for several generations, is no justification for postponing the study . . . . Our difficulties of the moment must always be dealt with somehow: but our permanent difficulties are difficulties of every moment. (Eliot 1949, p. 5)

How could the information summarized in this volume be used to prevent schizophrenia? First, we may find that we have already unknowingly decreased one form of schizophrenia—that associated with Rh incompatibility. Yet, despite the fact that we have had the ability to prevent Rh-incompatible pregnancies from developing into Rh HDN for a number of years, Rh HDN remains a significant contributor to infant morbidity and mortality in the United States (Chavez et al. 1991). Chavez and colleagues point out that there are a number of reasons for the continued presence of Rh HDN, including failure to use anti-D gamma globulin prophylaxis after an induced or spontaneous abortion, after an ectopic pregnancy, and after transfusion of Rh-positive blood products and failure to use it antenatally (to prevent small amounts of fetal blood that enter the mother's circulation from sensitizing her). The recognition that there may be an association between Rh incompatibility and schizophrenia should fuel the argument for a more concerted effort toward Rh prophylaxis. The pregnant women in the study by Hollister and colleagues (1996; see Chapter 8, this volume) were selected in part because they were thought to be at risk for giving birth to infants with HDN, and their pregnancies therefore may not be representative of pregnancies in general.

Until the results of Hollister et al. are replicated in a more representative sample of pregnancies, it is difficult to determine the proportion of schizophrenia cases that might be attributable to Rh incompatibility. In many Asian countries, for instance, where Rh-negative individuals are extremely rare, Rh incompatibility probably makes little or no contribution to schizophrenia. In the United States, however, 10% of Caucasian pregnancies are Rh incompatible. If even 1% of schizophrenia is attributable to Rh incompatibility, and schizophrenia costs the United States $65 billion in direct and indirect dollars per year (Wyatt et al. 1995), the annual cost of Rh-incompatible pregnancies leading to schizophrenia for this nation is roughly $650 million, not including the costs from nonschizophrenic disorders. In contrast, the cost of administering anti-D gamma globulin following delivery in an Rh-incompatible pregnancy is less than $15 (Pharmacy, Fairfax Hospital [Fairfax, Virginia], telephone communication, January 29, 1996).

The finding that severe nutritional deficiencies during the first trimester of pregnancy can lead to schizophrenia in the offspring raises the intriguing question of the responsible factor or factors. Although every attempt must be made to prevent famines of the kind that occurred during the Dutch Hunger Winter, doing so is more of a political and social science problem than a medical one. Nevertheless, if depletion of a specific nutritional factor is found to cause schizophrenia, there might be many situations in which that nutrient could be provided to pregnant women when calories could not. Furthermore, finding that such a severe nutritional deficiency is capable of causing schizophrenia suggests that other non-famine-related nutritional deficiencies might also be associated with other forms of schizophrenia. Links have been established between a number of vitamin deficiencies and various illnesses, including the well-publicized association between maternal folate and spina bifida. Studies by Mills and colleagues (1995) indicate that there is an additional interaction between the genetic defect of homocysteine metabolism and low maternal folate in producing neural tube defects. Once the association between low folate and neural tube defects was demonstrated by epidemiological studies, designed experiments were able to show that folate supplements could reduce neural tube defects (Czeizel and Dudas 1992; Medical Research Council Vitamin Study Research Group 1991); as a result, it has recently been recommended that all women of childbearing age take supplemental folate (Centers for Disease Control and Prevention 1995). Other nutritional factors could similarly be provided as preventive measures for schizophrenia.

Although studies searching for an association between second-trimester infection with influenza and development of schizophrenia in the offspring have had mixed results (Wyatt et al. 1996), the association has been replicated often enough to be intriguing; furthermore, it is consistent with neurodevelopmental models of schizophrenia. It is remarkable, given the nature of the available data, that the original finding (Mednick et al. 1988) has been replicated in at least 10 subsequent studies (Wright and Murray 1995; Wyatt et al. 1996). At what point do we decide that there is sufficient evidence that influenza infection during the second trimester is a risk factor for schizophrenia in a woman's offspring and consider a more active immunization program for women of childbearing age? Most importantly, should such a program be attempted before it is determined whether immunization itself could trigger a reaction in an already pregnant woman, with the possibility of subsequently producing schizophrenia in her offspring? Fortunately, even if such a triggered reaction were possible, it should be preventable. Given that the association between influenza and schizophrenia applies only during the second trimester, screening women of childbearing age for pregnancy prior to immunization would lessen morbidity while adding little to the cost of the immunization program.

Shifting the Paradigm

Although there is only weak evidence of an ongoing, active process beyond the initial phases of schizophrenia, there is much better evidence that early and perhaps sustained intervention with antipsychotic medications decreases some of the long-term morbidity associated with schizophrenia. As the authors of these chapters have pointed out, there is also evidence that some events during pregnancy place the fetus at risk for developing schizophrenia. Taken together, these two concepts should spark optimism that the future will bring advances in primary and secondary prevention; both have the real potential to decrease the morbidity and perhaps the incidence of schizophrenia. It may well be that some of the effort now going into research on rehabilitation and improved treatments might become less necessary if greater effort were directed at research related to secondary and especially primary prevention. Such a shift in policy, however, would also require a shift in thinking about schizophrenia. That shift would require both researchers and policy makers to seriously consider that schizophrenia may not be inevitable and that, even when the disorder is present, intervention may mean more than palliation.

References

Akbarian S, Kim J, Potkin S, et al: Gene expression for glutamic acid decarboxylase is reduced without loss of neurons in prefrontal cortex of schizophrenics. Arch Gen Psychiatry 25:258–266, 1995

Antonarakis SE, Blouin JL, Pulver AE, et al: Schizophrenia susceptibility and chromosome 6p24–22 (letter). Nat Genet 11:235–236, 1995

Bleuler M: The Schizophrenic Disorders: Long-Term Patient and Family Studies. Translated by Clemens SM. New Haven, CT, Yale University Press, 1978

Bogerts B: Recent advances in the neuropathology of schizophrenia. Schizophr Bull 19:431–445, 1993

Bunn H: Disorders of hemoglobin, in Harrison's Principles of Internal Medicine. Edited by Isselbacher K, Braunwald E, Wilson J, et al. New York, McGraw-Hill, 1994, pp 1734–1743

Carter M, Watts C: Possible biological advantages among schizophrenic's relatives. Br J Psychiatry 118:453–460, 1971

Catalano LW Jr, Sever JL: The role of viruses as causes of congenital defects. Annu Rev Microbiol 25:255–282, 1971

Centers for Disease Control and Prevention: Knowledge and use of folic acid by women of childbearing age—United States, 1995. JAMA 274:1190, 1995

Chavez GF, Mulinare J, Edmonds LD: Epidemiology of Rh hemolytic disease of the newborn in the United States. JAMA 265:3270–3274, 1991

Clements G, Galbraith D, Taylor K: Coxsackie B virus infection and onset of childhood diabetes. Lancet 346:221–223, 1995

Couch RB: Advances in influenza virus vaccine research. Ann N Y Acad Sci 685:803–812, 1993

Coyle J, Puttfacken P: Oxidative stress, glutamate, and neurodegenerative disorders. Science 262:695–700, 1993

Czeizel A, Dudas I: Prevention of the first occurrence of neural-tube defects by periconceptional vitamin supplementation. N Engl J Med 327:1832–1835, 1992

Davis J: Maintenance therapy and the natural course of schizophrenia. J Clin Psychiatry 11:18–21, 1985

Denicoff KD, Rubinow DR, Papa MZ, et al: The neuropsychiatric effects of treatment with interleukin-2 and lymphokine-activated killer cells. Ann Intern Med 107:293–300, 1987

Desjardins L, Blajchman M, Chintu C, et al: The spectrum of ABO hemolytic disease in the newborn infant. J Pediatr 95:447–449, 1979

Dohrenwend BP, Levav I, Shrout PE, et al: Socioeconomic status and psychiatric disorders: the causation-selection issue. Science 255:946–952, 1992

Eaton WW: Update on the epidemiology of schizophrenia. Epidemiol Rev 13:320–328, 1991

Eaton WW, Hayward C, Ram R: Schizophrenia and rheumatoid arthritis: a review. Schizophr Res 6:181–192, 1992

Ehrentheil O: Common medical disorders rarely found in psychotic patients. Arch Neurol Psychiatry 77:178–186, 1957

Eliot TS: Christianity and Culture. New York, Harcourt Brace, 1949

Erlenmeyer-Kimling L: Mortality rates in offspring of schizophrenic parents and a physiological advantage hypothesis. Nature 220:798–800, 1968

Feney GH: Juvenile-onset diabetes and schizophrenia? Lancet 2:1214–1215, 1989

Gresser I, Halstead S: Serologic response to Far East influenza. Arch Intern Med 103:590–592, 1959

Hollister JM, Laing P, Mednick SA: Rhesus incompatibility as a risk factor for schizophrenia in male adults. Arch Gen Psychiatry 53:19–24, 1996

Horuk R, Chitnis CE, Darbonne WC, et al: A receptor for the malarial parasite *Plasmodium vivax:* the erythrocyte chemokine receptor. Science 261:1182–1184, 1993

Huxley J, Mayr E, Osmond H: Schizophrenia as a genetic morphism. Nature 204:220–221, 1964

Jakob H, Beckmann H: Prenatal developmental disturbances in the limbic allocortex in schizophrenics. J Neural Transm 65:303–326, 1986

Jamison D: Disease control priorities in developing countries, in Disease Control Priorities in Developing Countries. Edited by Jamison D, Moseley W, Measham A, et al. New York, Oxford University Press, 1993, pp 3–34

Knight JG: Possible autoimmune mechanisms in schizophrenia. Integrative Psychiatry 3:134–143, 1985

Knight JG, Knight A, Ungvari G: Can autoimmune mechanisms account for the genetic predisposition to schizophrenia? Br J Psychiatry 160: 533–540, 1992

Kohn M: The interaction of social class and other factors in the etiology of schizophrenia. Am J Psychiatry 133:177–180, 1976

Kosower NS, Gerad L, Goldstein M, et al: Constitutive heterochromatin of chromosome 1 and Duffy blood group alleles in schizophrenia. Am J Med Genet 60:133–138, 1995

Liberman R, Corrigan P: Designing new psychosocial treatments for schizophrenia. Psychiatry 56:238–253, 1993

Lynberg MC, Khoury MJ, Lu X, et al: Maternal flu, fever, and the risk of neural tube defects: a population-based case-control study. Am J Epidemiol 140:244–255, 1994

Marzek P, Haggerty R: Reducing Risks for Mental Disorders: Frontiers for Prevention Intervention Research. Washington, DC, National Academy Press, 1994

McGuire W, Hill AV, Allsopp CE, et al: Variation in the TNF-alpha promoter region associated with susceptibility to cerebral malaria. Nature 371:508–510, 1994

Medical Research Council Vitamin Study Research Group: Prevention of neural tube defects: results of the Medical Research Council Vitamin Study. Lancet 338:131–137, 1991

Mednick SA, Machon RA, Huttunen MO, et al: Adult schizophrenia following prenatal exposure to an influenza epidemic. Arch Gen Psychiatry 45:189–192, 1988

Mills JL, McPartlin JM, Kirke PN, et al: Homocysteine metabolism in pregnancies complicated by neural-tube defects. Lancet 345:149–151, 1995

Moises HW, Yang L, Kristbjarnarson H, et al: An international two-stage genome-wide search for schizophrenia susceptibility genes. Nat Genet 11:321–324, 1995

Molholm H: Hyposensitivity to foreign protein in schizophrenic patients. Psychiatr Q 16:565–571, 1942

Mortensen P: The occurrence of cancer in first admitted schizophrenic patients. Schizophr Res 12:185–194, 1994

Mourant A, Kopec A, Domaniewska-Sobczak K: Blood Groups and Diseases: A Study of Associations of Disease With Blood Groups and Other Polymorphisms. New York, Oxford University Press, 1978

Murphy B, Nelson D, Wright P, et al: Secretory and systemic immunological response in children infected with live attenuated influenza A virus vaccines. Infect Immun 36:1102–1108, 1982

Nelson J, Huges K, Smith A, et al: Maternal-fetal disparity in HLA class II alloantigens and the pregnancy-induced amelioration of rheumatoid arthritis. N Engl J Med 329:466–471, 1993

Poltorak M, Khoja I, Hemperly J, et al: Disturbances in cell recognition molecules (N-CAM and L1 antigen) in the CSF of patients with schizophrenia. Exp Neurol 131:266–272, 1995

Prescott CA, Gottesman II: Genetically mediated vulnerability to schizophrenia. Psychiatr Clin North Am 16:245–267, 1993

Raff M, Barres B, Burne J, et al: Programmed cell death and the control of cell survival: lessons from the central nervous system. Science 262: 695–700, 1993

Saha N, Tay J, Tsoi W, et al: Association of Duffy blood group with schizophrenia in Chinese. Genet Epidemiol 7:303–305, 1990

Schwab SG, Albus M, Hallmayer J, et al: Evaluation of a susceptibility gene for schizophrenia on chromosome 6p by multipoint affected sibpair linkage analysis. Nat Genet 11:325–327, 1995

Shiota K: Neural tube defects and maternal hyperthermia in early pregnancy: epidemiology in a human embryo population. Am J Med Genet 12:281–288, 1982

Stein Z, Susser M, Saenger G, et al (eds): Famine and Human Development: The Dutch Hunger Winter of 1944–1945. New York, Oxford University Press, 1975

Straub RE, MacLean CJ, O'Neill FA, et al: A potential vulnerability locus for schizophrenia on chromosome 6p24–22: evidence for genetic heterogeneity. Nat Genet 11:287–293, 1995

Strohman R: Epigenesis: the missing beat in biotechnology? Biotechnology (NY) 12:156–164, 1994

Susser ES, Lin SP: Schizophrenia after prenatal exposure to the Dutch Hunger Winter of 1944–45. Arch Gen Psychiatry 49:983–988, 1992

Susser ES, Neugebauer R, Hoek HW, et al: Schizophrenia after prenatal famine: further evidence. Arch Gen Psychiatry 53:25–31, 1996

Vinogradov S, Gottesman II, Moises HW, et al: Negative association between schizophrenia and rheumatoid arthritis. Schizophr Bull 17: 669–678, 1991

Waddington JL: Schizophrenia: developmental neuroscience and pathobiology. Lancet 341:531–536, 1993

Waddington JL, Youssef HA, Kinsella A: Sequential cross-sectional and 10-year prospective study of severe negative symptoms in relation to duration of initially untreated psychosis in chronic schizophrenia. Psychol Med 25:849–857, 1995

Wang S, Sun CE, Walczak CA, et al: Evidence for a susceptibility locus for schizophrenia on chromosome 6pter–p22. Nat Genet 10:41–46, 1995

Wegmann T, Lin H, Guilbert L, et al: Bidirectional cytokine interactions in the maternal-fetal relationship: is successful pregnancy a TH2 phenomenon? Immunol Today 14:353–356, 1993

Weinberger DR: Premorbid neuropathology in schizophrenia (letter). Lancet 2:445, 1988

White N, Breman J: Malaria and babesiosis, in Harrison's Principles of Internal Medicine. Edited by Isselbacher K, Braunwald E, Wilson J, et al. New York, McGraw-Hill, 1994, pp 887–895

Wiederkehr F: Analysis of cerebrospinal fluid proteins by electrophoresis. J Chromatogr 569:281–296, 1991

Wilson AG, Duff GW: Genetic traits in common diseases (editorial). BMJ 310:1482–1483, 1995a

Wilson AG, Duff GW: Tumor necrosis factor (letter). Lancet 345:649, 1995b

Wright P, Murray RM: Prenatal influenza, immunogens and schizophrenia, in The Neurodevelopmental Basis of Schizophrenia. Edited by Waddington J, Buckley PF. Austin, TX, RG Landes, 1995, pp 43–59

Wyatt R: Science and psychiatry, in Comprehensive Textbook of Psychiatry, IV. Edited by Kaplan H, Sadock B. Baltimore, MD, Williams & Wilkins, 1985, pp 2016–2027

Wyatt RJ: Neuroleptics and the natural course of schizophrenia. Schizophr Bull 17:325–351, 1991

Wyatt R: Antipsychotic medication and the long-term course of schizophrenia: therapeutic and theoretical implications, in Contemporary Issues in the Treatment of Schizophrenia. Edited by Shriqui C, Nasrallah H. Washington, DC, American Psychiatric Press, 1995a, pp 385–410

Wyatt R: Early intervention for schizophrenia: can the course of the illness be altered? Biol Psychiatry 38:1–3, 1995b

Wyatt R: Neurodevelopmental abnormalities and schizophrenia: a family affair. Arch Gen Psychiatry 53:11–18, 1996

Wyatt R, Alexander R, Egan M, et al: Schizophrenia, just the facts: what do we know, how well do we know it? Schizophr Res 1:3–18, 1988

Wyatt R, Henter I, Leary M, et al: An economic evaluation of schizophrenia—1991. Soc Psychiatry Psychiatr Epidemiol 30:196–205, 1995

Wyatt R, Apud J, Potkin S: New directions in the prevention and treatment of schizophrenia: a biological perspective. Psychiatry 59:357–370, 1996

Index

*Page numbers printed in **boldface** type refer to tables or figures.*